Dangerous Sex Offenders

*A Task Force Report of the
American Psychiatric Association*

Dangerous Sex Offenders

A Task Force Report of the
American Psychiatric Association

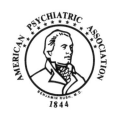

Published by the American Psychiatric Association
Washington, DC

Note: The authors have worked to ensure that all information in this book concerning drug dosages, schedules, and routes of administration is accurate as of the time of publication and consistent with standards set by the U.S. Food and Drug Administration and the general medical community. As medical research and practice advance, however, therapeutic standards may change. For this reason and because human and mechanical errors sometimes occur, we recommend that readers follow the advice of a physician who is directly involved in their care or the care of a member of their family.

The findings, opinions, and conclusions of this report do not necessarily represent the views of the officers, trustees, all members of the task force, or all members of the American Psychiatric Association. The views expressed are those of the authors of the individual chapters. Task force reports are considered a substantive contribution of the ongoing analysis and evaluation of problems, programs, issues, and practices in a given area of concern.

Manufactured in the United States of America on acid-free paper

First Edition

02   01   00   99   4   3   2   1
American Psychiatric Association
1400 K Street, N.W., Washington, DC   20005

Library of Congress Cataloging-in-Publication Data
Sexually dangerous offenders : A Task Force report of the American
   Psychiatric Association. — 1st ed.
      p.   cm.
   "The American Psychiatric Association, Task Force on Sexually
Dangerous Offenders"—P. preceding t.p.
   Includes bibliographical references and index.
   ISBN 0-89042-280-X
   1. Sex offenders—Mental health services.   2. Sex offenders—Legal
status, laws, etc.—United States.   3. Sex offenders—
Rehabilitation—United States.   I. American Psychiatric
Association.   Task Force on Sexually Dangerous Offenders.
   [DNLM: 1. Sex Offenses—United States legislation.   2. Sex
Offenses—psychology.   3. Sex Offenses—prevention & control—United
States.   4. Dangerous Behavior.   W 795 S5187 1999]
RC560.S47S5   1999
616.85'83—dc21
DNLM/DLC
for Library of Congress   98-50587
                                                                      CIP

British Library Cataloguing in Publication Data
A CIP record is available from the British Library.

Contents

Preface

This Task Force was created in response to the passage of statutes designed to civilly commit sex offenders to mental hospitals after they have served their entire prison sentences. These "sexual predator" statutes emerged in the context of some offenders committing heinous crimes against women and children after serving sentences for similar crimes. The current social milieu has also been characterized as emphasizing the retributive goals of punishment in contrast to the rehabilitative goals. The public seems to be demanding that sex offenders never recidivate and declaring that any method of incarceration or deterrence is acceptable. California recently passed legislation making surgical or chemical castration a requirement for parole of sex offenders. This kind of involuntary and intrusive treatment would have been unacceptable a few years ago. Some states have reactivated and modified their older "sexual psychopath" legislation. The "predator" statutes are different in some important ways from the older and largely repealed legislation that generally permitted hospitalization of "sexual psychopaths" in lieu of incarceration.

These developments have raised concerns among inmates subject to this type of confinement as well as among psychiatrists who are responsible for providing their treatment. As the Task Force began its deliberations it soon became clear that, except for a few dedicated researchers and clinicians, many psychiatrists were unfamiliar with the fundamentals of the assessment and treatment of sex offenders. Ignorance was coupled with fear of liability should the offender recidivate. Some of the concerns for the profession were clinical and others were policy considerations. For example:

- Is the "mental abnormality" requirement that includes antisocial personality disorder and other disorders not included in DSM a sufficient basis for the mental illness requirement of long-term civil commitment?
- Is pedophilia a mental disorder that justifies involuntary civil commitment?
- Are there current effective treatments for sex offenders in general or for specific subgroups?
- Are treatment and assessment of sex offenders readily available throughout the country?
- Does evaluation of sex offenders require special knowledge and techniques?
- Why is the literature on recidivism so conflicting or unclear? Are the "predator" statutes a legitimate effort to provide treatment or merely a pretext for preventive detention?
- Do any treatments decrease recidivism in a predictable fashion?
- Is involuntary civil commitment at the end of a penal sentence an appropriate legal remedy for offenders deemed likely to recidivate?

The Task Force has reviewed the literature on diagnoses, treatment, and recidivism and has attempted to provide a summary of that literature along with more comprehensive bibliographies for readers who may wish to pursue these topics in greater depth. Some of the policy questions are difficult and have not received much discussion in the literature. We have tried to identify those areas and to introduce some approaches that are consistent with American Psychiatric Association ethical guidelines and policy statements. We have also summarized the legal history of sexual psychopath and sexual predator legislation as well as the judicial reviews of this legislation. The U.S. Supreme Court in June 1997 held that these statutes were constitutional in the case of *Kansas v. Hendricks*, and a number of states have adopted or are considering similar statutes.

Although sexual predator statutes have withstood a constitutional challenge, they may not be the best approach to this complicated social and political problem. The statutes raise fundamental questions about the nature and purpose of civil commitment by their broad definitions of mental abnormality and confinement beginning only after completion of full prison terms. As a result of this decision, treatment of and release decisions regarding sex offenders will become a focus of attention for both correctional and mental health programs.

CHAPTER 1

Epidemiology of Sex Offenders and Mental Disorders Related to Sexual Behaviors

Human sexual behavior is diverse and is influenced by culture. In addition to the obvious role that sexual behavior plays in the preservation of the species, its major functions for human beings are related to bonding, expressing emotions between individuals, and recreation. Cross-cultural studies show wide diversity in what may be considered acceptable sexual behavior. However, some types of socially unacceptable sexual behavior are classified as unwanted conduct in every society. In the United States, sex offenses are generally defined by state and federal statutes and thus vary from jurisdiction to jurisdiction. Changing sexual mores are not always followed by new legislation, and this situation may result in the continuing presence of "blue laws" that reflect values of the past. These laws are generally not actively prosecuted or enforced. Criminal sexual behavior may be predicated on various factors such as consent, age, kinship, type of activity, gender of the partner, use of force, or location of the activity. Thus the same behavior may or may not be defined as criminal depending on the context.

Gebhard and colleagues offered a useful definition of sex offenders—tied to the legal definition of sex offenses—in 1967: "A sex offender is a person who has been legally convicted as the result of an overt act, committed by him for his own immediate sexual gratification, which is contrary to the prevailing sexual mores of the society in which he lives and/or is legally punishable."[1] Gebhard et al. also distinguish between sex offenders and sexually deviant individuals, who commit the same acts but have never been convicted in connection with their behavior.

Because this broad definition is linked to the criminal code, it can encompass such offenses as consensual sexual intercourse with a 15-year-old female by a 19-year-old male or homosexual conduct between consenting adults. It is therefore possible to have endless debates about the proper relationship between criminal prohibitions and prevailing sexual mores, especially if the society reflects heterogeneous sexual practices. However, for purposes of this report, the controversial aspects of criminalization of sex offenses are tangential to the much narrower category of offenses that are most pertinent to the work of the Task Force: 1) all nonconsensual sexual behavior, including rapes, other sexual assaults, touchings, and exposures, and 2) sexual behavior involving young children, even if it is consensual. For the most part, such behaviors are socially disapproved and criminally punishable in all societies, although some cultural variation arises at the margins both for nonconsensual behavior (e.g., the line between acceptable self-expression and indecent exposure) and for offenses involving minors (e.g., what the "age of consent" should be under statutory rape laws). Aside from these inevitable line-drawing problems, though, there is a general consensus about the types of sexual conduct that are regarded as sexually dangerous, and these are the behaviors that are addressed in this report.

It is best to begin by commenting on the frequency with which sex offenses are committed and the rates of offenders among population groups. Studies have been done in an attempt to differentiate between the number of crimes that have actually occurred and the number of crimes reported. In 1990 over 683,000 rapes were reported. It is noteworthy that only about one-third of these are reported to law enforcement agencies. The National Victim Center, after calculating how many victims would not discuss their rape even in an anonymous situation, estimated that the real rate might have been as high as 2 million.[2] That year the FBI reported that rapes were increasing four times faster than any other crime.[3] In 1994 the offense distribution of state prisoners showed that 88,000 of 906,000—or 9.7% of all prisoners—were incarcerated for violent sex offenses.[4] The United States has a rape rate four times higher than that of Germany, 13 times higher than that of Britain, and 20 times higher than that of Japan.[5] The National Victim Center survey estimated that 12 million women have been raped at some time in their lives. Sixty-one percent were under 18 at the time of their assault and 30% were under 11.

In 1995 the number of forcible rapes reported to the police nationwide was 97,460, the lowest total since 1989. The highest rate of forcible rape recorded by law enforcement agencies since 1976 was in 1992: 84 per 100,000 women or about 1 forcible rape for every 1,200 women. By 1995 the rate had decreased more than 14% to 72 per 100,000 women, or about 1 forcible rape for every 1,400 women. In 1995 law enforcement agencies reported that about half of all forcible rapes reported to law enforcement were cleared by arrest—representing an estimated 34,650 arrests for forcible rape. There were an additional 94,500 arrests for other sex offenses, including "statutory rape and offenses against chastity, common decency and morals." The per capita rate of arrest for forcible rape or sexual assault in 1995, 50.3 per 100,000 residents, was the same as in 1993.[6]

Federal statistical data sets on arrested or convicted persons, including the Uniform Crime Reports, National Judicial Reporting Program, and National Corrections Reporting Program, show a remarkable similarity in the characteristics of those categorized as rapists: 99 in 100 are male, 6 in 10 are white, and the average age is in the early 30s.

In 1992 an estimated 21,655 felony defendants nationwide were convicted of rape; 8 in 10 pleaded guilty. More than two-thirds of convicted rape defendants received a prison sentence. For rape defendants sentenced to prison, the average term imposed was just under 14 years. About 2% of convicted rapists received life sentences. Since 1980 the average annual growth rate of prisoners has been about 7.6%. The number of prisoners sentenced for violent sexual assault other than rape increased by an annual average of nearly 15%—faster than any other category of violent crime and faster than all other categories except drug trafficking.

The average sentence of convicted rapists released from state prison has remained stable at about 10 years, but the average time served has increased from about 3.5 years to about 5 years. For sexual assault the average sentence has been 6.5 years and the average time served increased by 6 months to just under 3 years. In two 3-year follow-ups of samples of felons placed on probation or released from prison, the Bureau of Justice Statistics found that rapists had a lower rate of rearrest for a new violent felony than most other categories of offenders convicted of violence. Yet rapists were more likely than others to be rearrested for a new rape.[7]

An estimated 18.6% of inmates serving time in state prisons in 1991 for violent crimes, or about 61,000 offenders nationwide, had been convicted of a crime against a victim under age 18. Two-thirds of all prisoners convicted of rape or sexual assault had committed their crime against a child. Three in 10 child victimizers reported they had committed their crimes against multiple victims. Three in four child victims of violence were female. For the vast majority of child victimizers in state prisons, the victim was someone they knew before the crime. A third had committed their crime against their own child. About half had a relationship with the victim as a friend, acquaintance, or relative other than offspring. About one in seven reported that the victim was a stranger to them.[8]

Psychopathology and Sexual Deviation

It is also possible to describe deviant and abnormal behavior apart from the legal definition of offenders. As with any abnormal behavior, many descriptive classifications and typologies have been proposed. One such classification is provided by clinical diagnosis focusing specifically on sexual deviation.

The question of whether all or some sexual offenders are mentally ill is complicated and controversial. Given the wide variety of behaviors and circumstances it is not surprising that there have been a variety of theories and proposed causes that range from biological to cultural. Great controversy has also arisen over the degree of control that sex offenders have over their behavior and thus what should be the appropriate societal response. Clearly some offenses can occur in the absence of any mental or physical disorder. Some sexual offenses occur in the context of more systemic physical or mental disorders that may affect behavior, such as mental retardation or traumatic brain injury. Others occur as part of primary sexual disorders—broadly categorized as paraphilias—such as pedophilia or exhibitionism, which can have obsessive or compulsive features. In addition, some offenders may have other mental disorders, ranging from disorders of psychotic proportions to the personality disorders, which may have a more indirect or derivative effect on specific sexual behavior.

When sexual behaviors become very different from the cultural norm, especially when they are harmful to others, clinicians attempt to better understand such behaviors by defining their characteristics. The definition and classification of deviant sexual behaviors have been very difficult because 1) they are committed by a small percentage of the population, 2) they are hidden by their participants, and 3) they are constantly modified by adaptation to changes in society.[9]

One commonly used classification concerns the so-called paraphilias. The fourth edition of the American Psychiatric Association's *Diagnostic and Statistical Manual of Mental Disorders* (DSM-IV) describes the essential features of a paraphilia to be

> recurrent, intense sexually arousing fantasies, sexual urges, or behaviors generally involving 1) nonhuman objects, 2) the suffering or humiliation of oneself or one's partner, or 3) children or other nonconsenting persons that occur over a period of at least six months (Criterion A). For some individuals, paraphilic fantasies or stimuli are obligatory for erotic arousal and are always included in sexual activity. In other cases, the paraphilic preferences occur only episodically (e.g., perhaps during periods of stress), whereas at other times the person is able to function sexually without

paraphilic fantasies or stimuli. The behavior, sexual urges or fantasies cause clinically significant distress or impairment in social, occupational, or other important areas of functioning (Criterion B).[10]

DSM-IV emphasizes that a paraphilia must be distinguished
from the nonpathological use of sexual fantasies, behaviors, or objects as a stimulus for sexual excitement in individuals without a
paraphilia. Fantasies, behaviors, or objects are paraphilic only
when they lead to clinically significant distress or impairment (e.g.,
are obligatory, result in sexual dysfunction, require participation
of nonconsenting individuals, lead to legal complications, or interfere with social relationships).[11]

The individual paraphilia (*para* indicating deviation) can be distinguished based on that to which the individual is attracted
(*philia*). Exhibitionism (exposure of genitals), fetishism (use of non-
living objects), frotteurism (touching and rubbing against a
nonconsenting person), pedophilia (focus on prepubescent children), sexual masochism (receiving humiliation or suffering), sexual sadism (inflicting humiliation or suffering), voyeurism
(observing sexual activity), transvestic fetishism (cross-dressing),
and paraphilia not otherwise specified (paraphilias that are less
frequently encountered) are all defined in DSM-IV. It is not uncom-
mon for individuals to have more than one paraphilia.[12]

There has been controversy regarding whether a small group of
rapists should be considered to have a paraphilia. Some specialists
within the field have concluded that the weight of scientific evidence supported the inclusion of some rapes as a paraphilia called
paraphilic coercive disorder. This category was intended for individuals with intense, repetitive urges of 6 months' duration to
commit rape, who had either acted on these urges or were disturbed by their presence. It is unclear what percentage of rapists
might be diagnosed as having a coercive paraphilic disorder, but
there is wide agreement that the percentage of rapists meeting
these criteria is small. It should be emphasized that paraphilic coercive disorder has never been listed as a diagnosis by the American
Psychiatric Association in its *Diagnostic and Statistical Manual of
Mental Disorders*.[13]

Rates of Psychopathology Among Offender Populations

As noted above, we lack reliable data on 1) actual rates of sexual offending (defined in legal terms) and 2) rates of sexual deviations (defined in clinical terms) in the general population. However, the more pertinent question for this report concerns the rates of sexual deviation (and other types of psychopathology) among identified sex offender populations, particularly correctional populations.

The research on the prevalence of mental illness among sex offenders has varied over time. The early studies from the 1930s to the 1950s showed a higher percentage of psychotic diagnoses and of course were dependent on the populations studied. It is a reasonable summary of the literature to state that although most sex offenders show traits of personality disorders and although there are subgroups representing the seriously mentally ill and developmentally disabled, most sex offenders do not show major psychiatric disorders. Data are less clear on the prevalence of alcoholism.

Figure 1–1 illustrates the self-reported complaints of individuals who appeared for assessments in 140 sexual treatment clinics in North America.[14]

There are many typologies of child molesters and rapists. None are solely diagnostically based. Typologies are developed with the hope that they will enhance the ability to predict behavior. The field has not yet developed to the point that this is feasible. The FBI is conducting research in an effort to distinguish between serial and solo rapists and between "escalators" and "nonescalators."[15,16] FBI typologies of child molesters include the following types:[17]

- **Regressed**—Immature, socially inept individuals who relate to children as peers. These individuals may be experiencing a brief period of low self-esteem and turn to their own children or other available juveniles.
- **Morally indiscriminate**—Antisocial individuals who use and abuse everything they touch. Their victims are chosen on the basis of vulnerability and opportunity and only coincidentally because they are children.

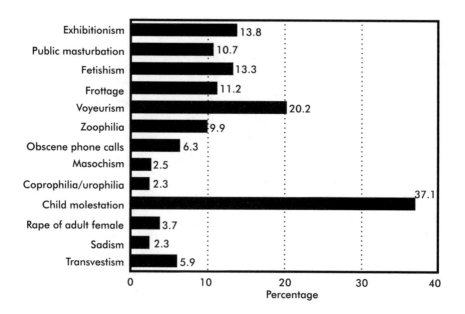

Figure 1–1.   Sexual behavior of 2,129 patients.
Source.   Data from G. Abel, personal communication, April 1998.

- **Sexually indiscriminate**—Referred to in the psychoanalytic literature as "polymorphous perverse," these individuals have vaguely defined sexual preferences and will experiment with almost any type of sexual behavior.
- **Inadequate**—Social misfits who may be developmentally disabled, psychotic, senile, or organically dysfunctional. These individuals rarely have contact with others and may see children as vulnerable objects with which to satisfy their sexual curiosity. They have been known to murder their victims. However, any type of molester is capable of murder in attempting to avoid detection.

Thus pedophilic behavior will have many potential diagnostic labels, ranging from no specific mental disorder to personality disorders, paraphilias, and other serious mental illnesses.

Although DSM-IV is silent on the issue of "compulsive sexual behavior," some researchers have organized their work around this concept. The term is generally meant to indicate excessive or uncontrolled behavior or sexual cognitions that lead to subjective distress or to social or occupational impairment or that have legal and financial consequences. Compulsive sexual behavior includes paraphilic and nonparaphilic behaviors. The latter include conventional sexual behaviors that have become excessive or uncontrolled. Coleman delineated five subtypes: 1) compulsive cruising and multiple partners, 2) compulsive fixation on an unobtainable partner, 3) compulsive masturbation, 4) compulsive multiple love relationships, and 5) compulsive sexuality within a relationship.[18] Only three or four studies have attempted to use this type of definition, and their samples are relatively small.[19–22]

In sum, the psychiatric nosology does not contribute in a systematic way to clinical understanding or treatment of sex offenders. Only the paraphilic diagnoses focus directly on psychopathological features of deviant sexual behavior, but these conditions appear to be absent in most offenders. In contrast, a significant number of sex offenders may have substance abuse or personality disorder diagnoses, but these conditions usually have little explanatory connection to the offender's sexual behavior. Unfortunately, however, concerned legislatures have sought to use the existence of a personality disorder per se as a basis for civil commitment of a sex offender. Thus the statutory category of "mental disorders" has been defined in a manner that bears no relationship to the usual moral and clinical criteria for criminal responsibility or to the usual predicates for compulsory psychiatric hospitalization or treatment.

References

1. Gebhard P, Gagnon J, Pomeroy W, et al: Sex Offenders: An Analysis of Types. New York, Bantam Books, 1967, p 9
2. Unsettling report on an epidemic of rape. Time, May 4, 1992, p 15
3. Salhotz E: Women under assault: sex crimes finally get the media's attention. Newsweek, July 16, 1990, p 23
4. Greenfeld L: Sex Offenses and Offenders: An Analysis of Data on Rape and Sexual Assault (NCJ-163392). Washington, DC, Bureau of Justice Statistics, 1997

5. Salhotz, *supra* note 2

6. Greenfeld, *supra* note 3

7. Greenfeld, *supra* note 3

8. Greenfeld L: Child Victimizers: Violent Offenders and Their Victims (NCJ-153258). Washington, DC, Bureau of Justice Statistics, 1996

9. Abel G: Paraphilias, in Comprehensive Textbook of Psychiatry/V, 5th Edition. Edited by Kaplan HI, Sadock BJ. Baltimore, MD, Williams & Wilkins, 1989, pp 1069–1085

10. American Psychiatric Association: Diagnostic and Statistical Manual of Mental Disorders, 4th Edition. Washington, DC, American Psychiatric Association, 1994, pp 522–523

11. *Id.* at 525

12. *Id.* at 523, 525

13. Abel, *supra* note 8, at 1079–1080

14. Abel G: Personal communication, April 1998

15. Warren J, Reboussin R, Hazelwood R, et al: Prediction of rapist type and violence from verbal, physical and sexual scales. Journal of Interpersonal Violence 6(1):55–67, 1991

16. Warren J, Hazelwood R, Reboussin R: Serial rape: the offender and his rape career, in Rape and Sexual Assault III: A Research Handbook. Edited by Burgess AW. New York, Garland, 1991, pp 76–102

17. Lanning K: Child Molesters: A Behavioral Analysis for Law Enforcement Officers Investigating Cases of Sexual Exploitation. Washington, DC, National Center for Missing and Exploited Children, 1986

18. Coleman E: Is your patient suffering from compulsive sexual behavior? Psychiatric Annals 22:320–325, 1992

19. Black D, Kehrberg L, Flumerfelt D, et al: Characteristics of 36 subjects reporting compulsive sexual behavior. Am J Psychiatry 154(2):243–249, 1997

20. Quadland MC: Compulsive sexual behavior: definition of a problem and an approach to treatment. J Sex Marital Ther 11:121–132, 1985

21. McConaghy N, Armstrong M, Blaszcynski A: Expectancy, covert sensitization, and imaginal desensitization in compulsive sexuality. Acta Psychiatr Scand 72:176–187, 1985

22. Kafka MP, Prentky R: A comparative study of nonparaphilic sexual addictions and paraphilias in men. J Clin Psychiatry 53:345–350, 1992

CHAPTER 2

Sexual Predator Commitment Laws: Legal Issues

Laws for the "special commitment" of sex offenders first appeared in the 1930s. Aimed at offenders believed to be at high risk for recidivism but at the same time good candidates for treatment, these laws provided for the indeterminate involuntary psychiatric hospitalization of persons found to be "sexual psychopaths."[1] The purpose of these laws was twofold: to "benefit sex offenders by curing them in perhaps a shorter time than they would serve as convicted criminals . . . [and to] protect society against premature release of dangerous offenders who had not been cured within the maximum period of incarceration available under a predicate criminal statute."[2]

By 1960, more than 25 states had enacted sex offender commitment laws, variously called "sexual psychopath" laws, "sexually dangerous persons" acts, and "mentally disordered sex offender" acts.[3] During the 1970s, however, these laws began to fall out of favor. The optimism of earlier decades that psychiatry held the cure to sexual psychopathy no longer shone so brightly. By 1990, all but 12 states and the District of Columbia had repealed their sexual psychopath commitment laws.[4] Moreover, of the jurisdictions with such laws still on the books in 1985, only six actually enforced them with any frequency.[5]

In the last 6 years, however, a number of states have resurrected the idea of special commitment for sex offenders. Washington, Wisconsin, Kansas, California, Arizona, Illinois, and North Dakota all have new commitment laws, and several other states have legislation pending.[6] Like their predecessors, sexual psychopath laws, these new laws allow for indeterminate commitment of offenders found to be, in today's parlance, "sexual predators." However, unlike many of the earlier laws—laws that provided for commitment as an alternative to prison—these new laws typically provide for commitment only after an offender has completed his or her criminal sentence. Thus, their primary purpose would appear to be incapacitative rather than therapeutic. No one has suggested that these laws reflect a renewed faith in the power of psychiatry to cure sex offenders.

History of Sexual Psychopath Laws

First-Generation Statutes: 1937–1990

Minnesota's "psychopathic personality" law, enacted in 1939, was typical of the first generation of sex offender commitment laws. It authorized the state to hospitalize anyone who met the statutory criteria of a "psychopathic personality":

> the existence in any person of such conditions of emotional instability or impulsiveness of behavior, or lack of customary standards of good judgment, or failure to appreciate the consequences of his acts, or a combination of any such conditions, as to render such a person irresponsible for his conduct with respect to sexual matters and thereby dangerous to other persons.[7]

Persons committed under the law remained confined until a special review board found them to be no longer in need of inpatient treatment and supervision, no longer dangerous to the public, and capable of making an acceptable adjustment to open society.[8]

Most of the early sexual psychopath laws (although not Minnesota's) reserved commitment for persons who had been convicted of a crime, typically a sex crime.[9] Some required only that the person be charged with a crime.[10] In five states, a person could be committed whether or not criminal charges had been brought.[11]

If the offender's commitment was triggered by a criminal conviction and was ordered in lieu of sentencing, then, in some states, the commitment served as a bar to further criminal proceedings or incarceration.[12] Other states allowed the offender to be returned to court for sentencing after completion of the commitment.[13] In a few states, offenders committed for a period less than the maximum sentence for the crime of conviction would be required to serve the remainder of such sentence upon release from the hospital.[14]

These early sexual psychopath commitment laws, by providing for hospitalization in lieu of imprisonment (at least initially), reflected a view that sex offenders were ill and that psychiatrists could cure them.[15] The American Bar Association, in commentary to its Criminal Justice/Mental Health Standards, observed that sexual psychopath legislation rested on six assumptions:

1. There is a specific mental disability called sexual psychopathy . . .;
2. Persons suffering from such a disability are more likely to commit serious crimes, especially dangerous sex offenses, than normal criminals;
3. Such persons are easily identified by mental health professionals;
4. The dangerousness of these offenders can be predicted by mental health professionals;
5. Treatment is available for the condition; and
6. Large numbers of persons afflicted with the designated disabilities can be cured.[16]

Although there was little to support these assumptions, sexual psychopath laws remained on the books for many years.

Movement Toward Repeal

During the 1970s and 1980s, laws for the special commitment of sex offenders came under attack. Positing that treatment for sexual psychopaths was ineffective, professional organizations such as the Group for the Advancement of Psychiatry (GAP)[17] and the American Bar Association's Committee on Criminal Justice Mental Health Standards,[18] as well as the President's Commission on Mental Health,[19] urged that these laws be repealed. GAP declared:

> *First and foremost, sex psychopath and sexual offender statutes can best be described as approaches that have failed.* The discrepancy between the promises in sex statutes and performances have rarely been resolved. . . . The notion is naive and confusing that a hybrid amalgam of law and psychiatry can validly label a person a "sex psychopath" or "sex offender" and then treat him in a manner consistent with a guarantee of community safety. The mere assumption that such a heterogeneous legal classification could define treatability and make people amenable to treatment is not only fallacious; it is startling.[20]
>
> Our position is that the experiment was a form of well intentioned but misguided intervention. Its dual goals have often remained in conflict. After a given passage of time an experiment needs evaluation in terms of its demonstrable benefits and liabilities. If the assessment of the statute in terms of achieving certain goals, for whatever reasons, leads to the conclusion that an experiment has not been successful, it should be halted.[21]

Even before the publication of the GAP report, courts in a few states had begun to take a dim view of sexual psychopath laws. In 1969, one court observed that " '[n]on-criminal' commitments of so-called dangerous persons have long served as preventive detention, but this function has been either excused or obscured by the promise that, while detained, the potential offender will be rehabilitated by treatment. Notoriously, this promise of treatment has served only to *bring an illusion of benevolence to what is essentially a warehousing operation for social misfits* [emphasis added]."[22]

Although the movement to repeal these laws was fueled primarily by disenchantment with the efficacy of treatment for sex offenders, in a few states, interestingly, repeal came about as a result of public concern over the premature release of offenders hospitalized as sexual psychopaths.[23] In 1976, James Ziglinski was convicted of several rapes and other offenses involving children in Wisconsin.[24] Under Wisconsin's Sex Crimes Act, Ziglinski was committed to the state's Central State Hospital.[25] His release in 1979—sooner than if he had gone to prison—outraged the public and prompted the Wisconsin legislature to repeal its act.[26]

By 1990, only 13 jurisdictions still had sexual psychopath laws in place, down from 28 in the 1960s.[27] Whether in a given state repeal came about as a result of a case like Ziglinski's or the lobbying efforts of professional associations, ultimately the demise of these laws can be attributed to a changing criminology in the United States—one in which rehabilitation has given way to retribution ("just deserts") as the paramount concern in criminal justice.

Criminal Justice in the Late 20th Century: Implications for the Disposition of Sex Offenders

For the first three-quarters of the 20th century, sentencing laws in the United States were generally indeterminate in nature.[28] Offenders facing incarceration typically were sentenced to potentially lengthy periods of confinement and placed in departments of "correction," where, in keeping with the "rehabilitative ideal,"[29] efforts were made to "change [the offender's] underlying personality and to make him safe to be returned to society."[30] Those offenders who showed promise for leading safe and productive lives in the community were considered for early release on parole. Those who were more recalcitrant in some cases served their entire sentences in confinement.[31] Laws for the special commitment of sexual psychopaths and other "defective delinquents" flourished during these years.

By the early 1980s, however, the philosophy of the criminal justice system in America had begun to change. Faced with high recidivism rates among paroled offenders, a growing disillusionment with rehabilitation, and concerns about disparity in treatment among offenders, states began to abandon indeterminate sentencing and special commitment laws in favor of laws that prescribed a fixed or presumptive penalty in every case—one that the offender would be required to serve in its entirety regardless of his or her behavior while incarcerated or prospects for success upon release.[32] To effect such reform without bringing about an explosion in the population of incarcerated offenders, however, lawmakers establishing determinate sentencing systems found it necessary to prescribe sentences that reflected the average period of time similarly situated offenders (i.e., those convicted of the same offense and having a similar criminal record) would have served had indeterminate sentencing not been abolished.[33] Thus, for example, if it were determined that under indeterminate sentencing in a given state second-degree murderers with one prior felony conviction historically had served on average 7 years in prison before release on parole (despite sentences ranging from 15 to 25 years and actual time served ranging from 3 to 25 years), then, with determinate sentencing, all second-degree murderers with one prior felony conviction would be sentenced to (and would be required to serve) 7 years.[34] Those who under indeterminate sentencing would have won early release on parole might spend a longer time confined under such a system, but those who would have failed to qualify for parole (because of their perceived "dangerousness") might complete their sentences and gain their freedom long before they would have under an indeterminate system. Ironically, it may be this hard reality of determinate sentencing—earlier release of some high-risk offenders—that accounts for the renewed interest nationally in schemes for the indeterminate commitment of sex offenders upon completion of sentence.

When Washington State enacted sentencing reform in 1981[35]—establishing a "presumptive sentence"[36] for every offense and eliminating discretionary parole—lawmakers prescribed a penalty of 5 years for first-degree rape,[37] roughly the average time that first-degree rapists in Washington had served before release on parole. Rapists sentenced to 5 years were required to serve the entire period in confinement but not a day longer. There was no parole to deny, and sentences could not be extended without violating constitutional ex post facto restrictions. The state was simply without authority to hold back those rapists who appeared at high risk for recidivism—at least not on criminal justice grounds. The question naturally arose, Might the state achieve preventive detention of these offenders on other grounds? Could the state keep sex offenders confined by means of civil commitment? As the legislature in Washington observed, the state's ordinary civil commitment laws would not do: "The Legislature finds that a small but extremely dangerous group of sexually violent predators exist who do not have a mental disease or defect that renders them appropriate for the existing involuntary treatment act. . . . The existing act, Chapter 71.05 RCW, is inadequate to address the risks to reoffend because during confinement these offenders do not have access to potential victims and therefore they will not engage in an overt act during confinement as required by the involuntary treatment act for continued confinement. The legislature further finds that the prognosis for curing sexually violent offenders is poor, the treatment needs of this population are very long, and the treatment modalities for this population are very different from the traditional treatment modalities for people appropriate for commitment under the involuntary treatment act."[38] If commitment were going to be possible, a special commitment law would have to be written.

Old Wine in New Bottles: The Sexual Predator Commitment Laws

Washington's sexual predator statute was prompted in large part by the case of Earl K. Shriner. On May 20, 1989, 2 years after completing a 10-year sentence for kidnapping and assaulting two teenage girls, Shriner raped a 7-year-old boy and cut off his penis.[39] In response to public outcry over the incident, the governor of Washington appointed a task force to study the problem and recommend "solutions."[40] The task force convened promptly and by the end of November 1989 submitted a report proposing an extensive package of legislation—the Community Protection Act—designed to protect the public from sex offenders.[41] The legislature passed the Community Protection Act on February 28, 1990.[42]

The Community Protection Act increased penalties for sex crimes by an average of 50%, extended postrelease supervision for certain sex offenders, and required convicted sex offenders to register with the police.[43] Most importantly, perhaps, this legislation established a new law for the civil commitment of persons found to be "sexually violent predators."[44]

Washington's sexual predator commitment law is different from many of the earlier sexual psychopath commitment laws in that under the Washington law, commitment is not intended as a substitute for punishment. The offender is subject to commitment only *after* serving his or her full prison term (or after being charged with a criminal offense and found to be incompetent to stand trial or not guilty by reason of insanity and no longer eligible for confinement).[45] Moreover, no showing need be made that the offender has committed a recent act of sexual violence. Indeed, there is no requirement that the offender have behaved inappropriately in any way since the crime for which the offender was originally charged.[46] All the state need show is that the offender is a "sexually violent predator": "a person who has been convicted of or charged with a crime of sexual violence and who suffers from a mental abnormality or personality disorder which makes the person likely to engage in predatory acts of sexual violence."[47] "Mental abnormality," as defined by the Washington law, is "a congenital or acquired condition affecting the emotional or volitional capacity which predisposes the person to the commission of criminal sexual acts."[48] "Personality disorder" is not defined.

The prosecuting attorney or attorney general may file a petition for commitment under the new law by alleging that a person 1) has been a) convicted of a sexually violent offense, b) found to have committed a sexually violent offense as a juvenile, c) charged with a sexually violent offense but determined to be incompetent to stand trial, or d) found not guilty by reason of insanity of a sexually violent offense; 2) is about to be released; and 3) appears to be a sexually violent predator.[49] Once a petition has been filed, the court must find whether there is probable cause to believe that the person is a sexually violent predator.[50] If probable cause is found, the person is taken into custody and evaluated by a mental health professional "deemed to be professionally qualified to conduct such an examination pursuant to rules developed by the Department of

Social and Health Services."[51] The person has the right to an additional examination by a qualified evaluator of his or her choosing.[52] An evaluator is provided at state expense if the person is indigent.[53] Within 45 days after the filing of the petition, a trial is held.[54] If the state proves beyond a reasonable doubt that the person is a sexually violent predator, the court will order the person "committed to the custody of the Department of Social and Health Services in a secure facility."[55] (The facility used at present is a unit within the walls of the state prison in Monroe, Washington.[56]) The law provides for confinement "until such a time as the person's mental abnormality or personality disorder has so changed that the person is safe to be at large."[57]

Washington's sexually violent predator law has been used as a model for legislation in other states. Indeed, laws in Wisconsin and Kansas are practically "carbon copies" of Washington's law. Terry Davis, Director of Quality Enhancement for Mental Health Programs in Kansas, has noted that the Kansas law has "all the problems" that the Washington statute has, in particular a contradiction right at the beginning: "It says people are untreatable, and then it says the program is for treatment."[58]

Legal Challenge to Washington's Sexually Violent Predator Law: *In re Young*

Washington's sexually violent predator law has been controversial from the outset. As the first of a new breed, the law has received extensive coverage in both the popular media and the professional literature. The *Puget Sound Law Review* devoted an entire issue (Spring 1992) to an examination of the "dichotomies raised by the statutes."[59] In addition to the obvious clinical and professional concerns—Is treatment effective? Do "sexual predators" merit such an allocation of psychiatric resources?—a fundamental legal question begs to be resolved: is the law constitutional? On August 6, 1993, the Washington Supreme Court, in the case *In re Young*,[60] ruled that it was. On August 25, 1995, a federal district court in Washington reversed the ruling.[61]

The Washington Supreme Court opinion joined two cases, those of Andre Young, a repeat rapist who had been committed pursuant to a petition filed one day prior to his release from prison, and Vance Cunningham, also a repeat rapist who had been released 4.5 months before the initiation of proceedings for his commitment. Young and Cunningham challenged their commitments on a number of constitutional grounds. First, they argued that the statute was unconstitutional because it violated the double jeopardy clause of the Fifth Amendment to the Constitution and the prohibition of ex post facto laws.[62] Observing that these protections apply only in criminal cases (or where the purpose or effect of the proceeding in question is punitive) and finding that the commitment here was civil in nature, the court rejected their claims: "Although the scheme here does involve an affirmative restraint, the civil commitment goals of incapacitation and treatment are distinct from punishment and have been so regarded historically."[63]

Second, Young and Cunningham argued that the Washington law violated substantive due process (as guaranteed by the Fourteenth Amendment) because it allowed the state to commit people without proving both mental illness and dangerousness. The court acknowledged that due process requires that both mental illness and dangerousness be shown (citing *Foucha v. Louisiana*, 112 S Ct 1780 [1991]), but it ruled that the Washington law was in accord. Observing that the law "inherently applies only to dangerous offenders"[64]—those "likely to engage in predatory acts of sexual violence"—the court declared that "there is no doubt that commitment is predicated on dangerousness under the statute."[65] With regard to the mental illness requirement, the court noted that the law called for proof of a "mental abnormality or personality disorder" and, quoting Brooks,[66] drew the following conclusion: "although 'mental abnormality' is not in the [DSM], . . . in using the concept of mental abnormality, the legislature has invoked a more generalized terminology that can cover a much larger variety of disorders. Some, such as the paraphilias, are covered in DSM-III-R; others are not. The fact that pathologically driven rape, for example, is not yet listed in DSM-III-R does not invalidate such a diagnosis. DSM is, after all, an evolving and imperfect document. Nor is it sacrosanct. Furthermore, it is in some areas a political document whose diagnoses are based in some cases on what the [American Psychiatric Association] leaders consider to be practical realities."[67]

The experts who testified at Young's and Cunningham's trials diagnosed "rape as paraphilia," within the category of "paraphilias not otherwise specified."[68] In addition, the state's expert in Young's trial diagnosed antisocial personality disorder.[69] Pointing to statutory language acknowledging that "sexually violent predators . . . have antisocial personality disorder features which are unamenable to existing mental illness treatment"[70] and that the "prognosis for curing sexually violent offenders is poor,"[71] Young and Cunningham argued that, regardless of the law's use of the terms *mental abnormality* and *personality disorder*, no real mental disorder was contemplated, "because treatment of sex offenders is impossible."[72] The court, however, disagreed, declaring that "the mere fact that an illness is difficult to treat does not mean that it is not an illness. . . . The legislature should not be admonished for its honest recognition of the difficulties inherent in treating those afflicted with the mental abnormalities causing the sex predator condition."[73] Although at no point did the court squarely address the incongruity in terminology—"mental abnormality or personality disorder" versus "mental illness"—it is implicit in the opinion that these terms were understood to be synonymous.

The petitioners also argued that their commitments were invalid because the state had not shown a recent overt act as evidence of their dangerousness. Such a showing must be made for ordinary civil commitment under Washington law.[74] Observing that for incarcerated offenders, "a requirement of a recent overt act under the statute would create a standard which would be impossible to meet,"[75] the court ruled that "where the individual is currently incarcerated no evidence of a recent overt act is required. However, where an individual has been released from confinement on a sex offense . . . and lives in the community immediately prior to the initiation of sex predator proceedings, the above rationale does not apply" and a recent overt act must be shown.[76] On this ground, the court overturned Cunningham's (but not Young's) commitment.

The petitioners also challenged the Washington law on procedural grounds, arguing that the equal protection principles of the

Fourteenth Amendment and of Washington State's Constitution required the state to accord sexual predators procedural protections equivalent to those accorded in the ordinary civil commitment process. The court, however, observed that "[e]qual protection does not require that all persons be dealt with identically, but it does require that a distinction have some relevance to the purpose for which the classification is made."[77] Noting that differential treatment is justified to some degree because of the special dangerousness of sexual predators,[78] the court rejected most of the petitioners' equal projection claims. For example, although persons subject to ordinary civil commitment proceedings enjoy a statutory right to remain silent, no such right need be accorded sexual predators, the court declared, because "the mental abnormalities or personality disorders involved with predatory behavior may not be immediately apparent. Thus, their cooperation with the diagnosis and treatment procedure is essential."[79] Some of the petitioners' equal protection claims, however, fared better. For example, the court ruled that the state had offered no justification for not considering less restrictive alternatives as required by civil commitment law and remanded Young's case for consideration of less restrictive alternatives.[80] The court, however, did not find the statute unconstitutional. Moreover, Young's remand did not result in his release.

In a dissenting opinion, Washington Supreme Court Justice Charles W. Johnson took issue with the majority's characterization of the statutory conditions "mental abnormality or personality disorder" as mental illnesses. Acknowledging the position of the Washington State Psychiatric Association (expressed in an amicus brief) that " 'mental abnormality' has no clinically significant meaning or recognized diagnostic use ... ,"[81] Justice Johnson concluded that these conditions do not constitute the kind of mental illness required for involuntary commitment. Indeed, Justice Johnson observed, "[t]he Statute, by its own terms applies specifically to individuals who do not have a mental disease or defect that renders them appropriate for the existing involuntary treatment act."[82]

Justice Johnson was particularly critical of the majority's han-

dling of the overt act requirement. "By reading in this new requirement [that a recent overt act be established for the commitment of
sexually violent predators who have been released from incarcera-
tion] the court creates two classes of persons under the same statute: those incarcerated versus those who are not. This is a
distinction without a difference. Immediately upon release, an individual must now commit an overt act to be incarcerated under
the statute whereas the day before release this same individual
could be committed without proof of an overt act. This new distinction is arbitrary, violating even a rational basis review."[83]

In conclusion, Justice Johnson warned that "by authorizing the
indefinite confinement in mental facilities of persons who are not
mentally ill, the statute threatens not only the liberty of certain sex
offenders, but the liberty of us all. By committing individuals
based solely on perceived dangerousness, this statute sets up an
Orwellian 'dangerousness court,' a technique of social control fundamentally incompatible with our system of ordered liberty guaranteed by the Constitution and contrary to the recent U.S. Supreme
Court decision in *Foucha v. Louisiana. . . .*"[84]

Disappointed with the majority's ruling in his case (but perhaps
heartened by Justice Johnson's dissent), Young appealed to the federal courts. On August 25, 1995, U.S. District Court Judge John C.
Coughenour overturned the Washington Supreme Court ruling,
declaring Washington's sexual predator commitment law constitutionally deficient.[85] Referencing a legislative history decrying the
powerlessness of the state under then-existing law to commit
"predators who had been judged not to have a mental illness or
mental disorder," Judge Coughenour concluded, "[t]his is not an
enactment designed to provide for the commitment of dangerous
mentally ill or mentally disordered persons. Rather, the statute tar-
gets persons with 'antisocial personality features.' " Quoting from
the U.S. Supreme Court's opinion in *Foucha v. Louisiana,* Judge
Coughenour reasoned that to allow the statute to stand "would
permit the state to hold indefinitely [persons] not mentally ill who
could be shown to have a personality disorder that may lead to
criminal conduct. The same would be true of any convicted criminal, even though he has completed his prison term. It would also

be only a step away from substituting confinements for dangerousness for our present system which, with only narrow exceptions and aside from permissible confinements for mental illness, incarcerates only those who are proved beyond reasonable doubt to have violated a criminal law."[86]

Because Washington was the first state to enact a law for the commitment of sexually violent predators, its law was the first of this new breed to be tested in the courts. Before long, however, state courts in both Wisconsin and Kansas had joined in the fray. The Wisconsin Supreme Court upheld its law; the Kansas Supreme Court declared its law unconstitutional.

State v. Post and State v. Oldakowski

The Wisconsin Supreme Court rendered its opinion in two cases decided jointly, *State v. Post* and *State v. Oldakowski*.[87] In upholding the law, the court heard and rejected essentially the same arguments Young had presented in his case in Washington State. Specifically, the court dismissed the notion that use of the term *mental disorder* rather than *mental illness* as the "mental condition component" of the commitment standard rendered the law constitutionally inadequate. "[T]here is no talismanic significance that should be given to the term 'mental illness,' "[88] the court declared. In addition, the court rejected the argument that due process was denied because treatment was not "a serious objective" of the commitment law. Pointing to language requiring the state to provide "control, care, and treatment" for those committed under the law, the court reasoned that treatment was a "bona fide goal of this statute."[89] Confronted with a professional literature divided on the question of whether sex offenders could be treated successfully, the court refused to recognize amenability to treatment as a prerequisite for commitment. Quoting from Justice Warren Burger's concurring opinion in the landmark civil commitment case *O'Connor v. Donaldson*,[90] the court observed that "[g]iven the present state of medical knowledge regarding abnormal human behavior and its treatment, few things would be more fraught with peril than to irrevocably condition a state's power to protect the mentally ill upon the providing of such treatment as will give them a realistic opportunity to be cured."[91]

In a stinging dissent, Justice Shirley S. Abrahamson slammed the majority position that because concepts of mental disorder are "fraught with medical and scientific uncertainties," courts should defer to legislative definitions: "[A] recognition that mental illness or the neologism 'mental condition component' may be defined in more than one way hardly suggests that mental illness can be defined howsoever the state pleases. If the constitutionally prescribed threshold of mental illness has no core meaning and can mean everything, then it means nothing. The *Foucha* case teaches that states are not free to define any deviancy they please as a mental illness and thereby commit to mental hospitals anyone who might fit their definition. Were there no limit on a state's substantive power to commit individuals, a state could civilly commit whole categories of criminal offenders such as intoxicated drivers merely by branding them deviant and designating them mentally disordered."[92]

In the Matter of Leroy Hendricks

Kansas's law for the commitment of sexually violent predators was tested in the case *In the matter of Leroy Hendricks.* In an opinion announced on March 1, 1996, the Kansas Supreme Court ruled the law unconstitutional, in violation of the Substantive due process clause of the Fourteenth Amendment to the U.S. Constitution. Noting that due process requires involuntary commitment to be based on a finding of both dangerousness and mental disorder, the court wrote, "[w]e find no support in the Act that a finding of mental illness is required. . . . K.S.A. 59–2901 states that sexually violent predators do not have a mental illness which 'renders them appropriate for involuntary treatment pursuant to the Treatment Act for Mentally Ill Persons defined in K.S.A. 59–2901 et seq.' The statute then contrasts sexually violent predators with 'persons appropriate for civil commitment under K.S.A. 59–2901 et seq.' in that they have 'antisocial personality features which are unamenable to existing mental illness treatment modalities.' By such language, the legislature recognizes that sexually violent predators are not mentally ill but, rather, have an 'antisocial personality feature' or a 'mental abnormality.' " "It is clear that the overriding concern of the legislature is to continue the segregation of sexual violent predators from the public. Treatment with the goal of reintegrating them into society is incidental, at best. The record reflects that treatment for sexually violent predators is all but nonexistent. The legislature concedes that sexually violent predators are not amenable to treatment under K.S.A. 59–2901 et seq. If there is nothing to treat . . . then there is no mental illness. In that light, the provisions of the act for treatment appear somewhat disingenuous."

In a concurring opinion, Justice Tyler C. Lockett observed, "[t]his case illustrates better than most that the process of judicial decision is often difficult to exercise. The hard fact is that sometimes we make decisions we do not like. We make them because they are right, right in the sense that the law and the Constitution as we see them compels [sic] the result." In a lengthy dissent, Justice Edward Larson challenged the "basic premise, the underlying reasoning, and the conclusion" of the majority. Seizing on language in the U.S. Supreme Court's opinion in *Addington v. Texas* that "[l]oss of liberty [in the context of civil commitment] calls for a showing that the individual suffers from something more serious than is demonstrated by idiosyncratic behavior," Justice Larson argued that the "mental infirmity" contemplated by the Kansas law, while perhaps not appearing in DSM, nonetheless is "an ailment of the mind, rather than mere 'idiosyncratic behavior. . . . ' " "[T]he fact that the legislature has chosen different definitions of mental ailments [than appear in DSM], and drawn the boundaries of what is a 'mental abnormality' in accordance with its limited purposes, is not an indictment of a statutory scheme, but rather is to its credit. It reflects that the legislature has narrowly tailored its statute to include only those persons presenting the precise danger the statute seeks to abate. DSM-IV defines classifications for purposes completely unrelated to protecting the public from sexually violent predators, and therefore it is of no moment that its classification of mental disorders differs from that adopted by the legislature." Finally, Justice Larson dismissed the notion that treatability should be a condition for commitment. "I would reject Hendricks' contention that the practical effect of the act is indeterminate incarceration and the statement of the majority [that] the treatment for sexually violent predators is all but nonexistent. The existence or extent of the specific care and treatment Hendricks has or will receive is not at issue here. It is clear that treatment is statutorily and constitutionally required."

New Challenges to the Sexual Psychopath Statutes: *In re Blodgett*

While courts in Washington State, Wisconsin, and Kansas grappled with the constitutionality of the new sexual predator commitment laws, Minnesota's psychopathic personality statute, enacted in 1939 (and discussed above), came under attack as well. The statute had first been challenged soon after its enactment and had been found constitutional by the U.S. Supreme Court (in the case *Minnesota ex rel. Pearson v. Probate Court of Ramsey County Minn.* [1940][93]). When in 1994 the statute was tested again (*In re Blodgett*[94]), the Minnesota Supreme Court was quick to rely on the U.S. Supreme Court's opinion in *Pearson*, ruling that nothing in the development of constitutional law since 1940 had rendered Minnesota's law invalid.[95]

Phillip Blodgett was a repeat sex offender who had nearly completed a 4-year prison term for raping a 16-year-old girl. Shortly before Blodgett's release, Dr. Richard Friberg evaluated Blodgett pursuant to the Minnesota Department of Corrections risk assessment and release procedures. Dr. Friberg notified the Washington County Attorney that based on his evaluation it appeared Blodgett met the conditions for commitment under the state's psychopathic personality statute. The Washington County Attorney filed a petition for Blodgett's commitment, and an initial hearing was conducted. Based on the testimony of five psychologists, four of whom stated that they felt Blodgett met the statutory definition of psychopathic personality, the court committed Blodgett to the Minnesota Security Hospital (MSH) and ordered the MSH staff to report back to the court within 60 days. In their report, the MSH staff concluded that Blodgett had antisocial personality disorder but recommended that he not be held in confinement as a psychopathic personality. At a subsequent hearing, Blodgett moved the court to dismiss on the ground that Minnesota's psychopathic personality statute was unconstitutional. The court denied Blodgett's motion, found that he continued to meet the criteria for commitment as a psychopathic personality, and ordered his retention in the hospital.

The court of appeals affirmed Blodgett's commitment,[96] and Blodgett petitioned the Minnesota Supreme Court for review. Blodgett argued that *Pearson* no longer was controlling in light of the U.S. Supreme Court's more recent decision in *Foucha v. Louisiana,* forbidding the psychiatric hospitalization of an insanity acquittee who no longer was mentally ill.[97] Blodgett argued that although he might be socially maladjusted, he was not mentally ill; therefore, *Foucha* forbade his commitment.[98]

The Minnesota court acknowledged that the term *psychopathic personality* did not appear in DSM and that the condition was not generally regarded by mental health professionals as a mental illness but declared, nonetheless, that it was an "identifiable and documentable violent sexually deviant condition or disorder" and not a mere social maladjustment.[99] Thus, the court ruled, it could provide the basis for a legitimate commitment.

Blodgett also argued that because the condition of psychopathic personality was untreatable, confinement was tantamount to lifelong preventive detention.[100] Despite the testimony of Dr. Michael Farnsworth, senior staff psychologist at the Minnesota Security Hospital, that any treatment Blodgett might receive would be a "sham" or "placebo,"[101] the court observed that it was not clear that treatment for the psychopathic personality never works.[102] The court also noted that even when treatment is problematic, so long as the commitment is for the *purpose* of treatment and is subject to periodic review, due process is provided.[103]

In a dissenting opinion, in which she was joined by two other justices, Justice Rosalie Wahl declared that the U.S. Supreme Court's opinion in *Foucha* "compels the conclusion that the Minnesota Psychopathic Personality Statutes . . . are violative of the Fourteenth Amendment and, therefore, unconstitutional."[104] Justice

Wahl reasoned that since Blodgett was not mentally ill, there could be no legitimate basis for his commitment to a psychiatric facility.[105]

Justice Wahl also found fault with the law's requirement that Blodgett prove he was no longer in need of inpatient treatment before he could be released.[106] If—as the very psychiatrists who were charged with treating Blodgett testified—there was no meaningful treatment for a psychopathic personality, how, Wahl asked, would Blodgett ever be able to win his release?[107] Indeed, why was he in a hospital?

Following *Blodgett,* Minnesota's sexual psychopath commitment law was challenged in federal court (*Nicolaison v. Erickson,* 65 F3d 109 [Sept. 7, 1995]), where with very little discussion the 8th Circuit Court of Appeals upheld the law, citing *Pearson* and *Blodgett.*

The Supreme Court Speaks: *Kansas v. Hendricks*

Given the impassioned debate these laws inspired and the inconsistent legal rulings from state to state, it was clear that the constitutionality of these laws would ultimately would have to be resolved by the U.S. Supreme Court. On June 23, 1997, the Court ruled, declaring in the Kansas case *Kansas v. Hendricks* (discussed above) that Kansas's Sexually Violent Predator Act was constitutional, at least as applied in the commitment of Leroy Hendricks.[108]

Writing for a five-justice majority, Justice Clarence Thomas rejected both of Hendricks's fundamental challenges to the law's constitutionality: 1) that by permitting his commitment upon a finding of "mental abnormality," the law violated the Constitution's substantive due process requirement that only persons found to be "mentally ill" were legitimate subjects for commitment; and 2) that by permitting commitment predicated on past conduct already adjudicated and for which he already had served a sentence, the law violated both the double jeopardy prohibition and the ban on ex post facto law making. Justice Thomas conceded that "[a] finding of dangerousness, standing alone, is ordinarily not a sufficient ground upon which to justify indefinite involuntary commitment . . . "—that "proof of some additional factor,

such as a 'mental illness' or 'mental abnormality' " would be necessary. But he flatly dismissed the notion that the mental condition in
question must be one classified or officially recognized by the mental health community. "[W]e have never required State legislatures
to adopt any particular nomenclature in drafting civil commitment
statutes. Rather, we have traditionally left to legislators the task of
defining terms of a medical nature that have legal significance."

Justice Thomas quickly disposed of Hendricks's double jeopardy
and ex post facto challenges as well, noting that these constitutional
protections are implicated only if a measure is punitive. Commitment
under the Kansas law is not punitive, Thomas declared, because it
"does not implicate either of the two primary objectives of criminal
punishment: retribution or deterrence." The act is not retributive, Justice Thomas wrote, because it affixes no culpability. "An absence of
the necessary criminal responsibility suggests that the state is not
seeking retribution for a past misdeed. Thus, the fact that the act may
be 'tied to criminal activity' is 'insufficient to render the statute punitive.' " Deterrence is not a feature of the Kansas law, Justice Thomas
reasoned, because "persons committed under the Act, by definition,
suffer from a 'mental abnormality' or a 'personality disorder' that
prevents them from exercising adequate control over their behavior . . . and [s]uch persons are therefore unlikely to be deterred by the
threat of confinement."

Finally, Justice Thomas addressed Hendricks's argument that
the Kansas law necessarily was punitive because it failed to offer
any legitimate treatment. Conceding the Kansas Supreme Court's
finding that "treatment for sexually violent predators is all but
nonexistent . . . [and] that sexually violent predators are not amenable to treatment under [the Kansas law]," Justice Thomas concluded, nonetheless, that the law was constitutional. "We have
never held that the Constitution prevents a state from civilly de-
taining those for whom no treatment is available, but who never-
theless pose a danger to others." Citing a U.S. Supreme Court
decision approving of pretrial detention of certain dangerous criminal defendants, Justice Thomas declared, "when accompanied by
proper procedures, incapacitation may be a legitimate end of the
civil law."

In a concurring opinion, Justice Anthony Kennedy agreed that Hendricks's commitment was constitutional, but he refused to accept the majority's conclusion that treatment need not be available. "If the object or purpose of the Kansas law had been to provide treatment but the treatment provisions were adopted as a sham or mere pretext, there would have been an indication of the forbidden purpose to punish." Justice Kennedy expressed particular concern about the legitimacy of "mental abnormality" as the predicate condition for commitment under the Kansas law. "[I]f it were shown that mental abnormality is too imprecise a category to offer a solid basis for concluding that civil detention is justified, our precedence would not suffice to validate it. . . . In this case, the mental abnormality—pedophilia—is at least described in the DSM-IV." Whether or not Justice Kennedy would approve the commitment of someone whose mental abnormality was not in DSM is not clear.

In a dissenting opinion, in which he was joined by three other justices, Justice Stephen Breyer identified three "obvious . . . resemblances between the Act's 'civil commitment' and traditional criminal punishments": 1) commitment "amounts to secure confinement" (akin to penal incarceration); 2) commitment is reserved for persons who have committed a criminal offense; and 3) commitment "imposes . . . confinement through the use of persons (county prosecutors), procedural guarantees (trial by jury, assistance of counsel, psychiatric evaluations), and standards ('beyond a reasonable doubt') traditionally associated with the criminal law." Noting, however, that "[t]hese obvious resemblances by themselves . . . are not legally sufficient to transform what the Act calls 'civil commitment' into a criminal punishment," Breyer declined to brand the law unconstitutional per se. Moreover, he refused "to consider whether the [Constitution] always requires treatment—whether, for example, it would forbid civil confinement of an untreatable mentally ill, dangerous person." Rather, Justice Breyer based his dissent on the failure of Kansas to provide treatment for Mr. Hendricks after arguing as a basis for his commitment that he had a condition for which treatment *was* available.[109] "[O]ne would expect a nonpunitively motivated legislature that confines because of a dangerous mental abnormality to seek to help the individual himself overcome that abnormality (at least insofar as professional treatment for the abnormality exists and is potentially helpful, as Kansas, supported by some groups of mental health professionals, argues is the case here . . .)." Moreover, Justice Breyer observed, "when a State believes that treatment does exist, and then couples that admission with a legislatively required delay of such treatment until a person is at the end of his jail term (so that further incapacitation is therefore necessary), such a legislative scheme begins to look punitive." Leaving open the possibility, however, that commitment under the law might be constitutional in a different case, Justice Breyer concluded, "[t]his analysis, rooted in the facts surrounding Kansas's failure to treat Hendricks, cannot answer the question whether the Kansas Act, as it now stands, and in light of its current implementation, is punitive towards people other than he. And I do not attempt to do so here."

Given that three justices joined in Justice Breyer's dissent, Justice Kennedy's vote with the majority served as the tiebreaker; thus, his concurring opinion may be read to limit the scope of the Court's decision in *Hendricks*. The decision, he wrote, "concerns Hendricks alone," suggesting that the case should not be read as a blanket endorsement of the Kansas statute. "Should a case arise involving an individual for whom treatment were shown to be a 'sham or mere pretext'—constitutionally unacceptable in Justice Kennedy's view—there is little doubt that Kennedy's stand with the majority would change, possibly tipping the balance of the Court."[110]

Treatability as a Prerequisite: Older Law

Although none of the recent court decisions—including the Supreme Court's in *Hendricks*—has explicitly found amenability to treatment or a proven treatment process to be a necessary condition for commitment, some older decisions have. In 1959, the Massachusetts Supreme Court ruled in *Commonwealth v. Page* that commitment under the Massachusetts Sexual Psychopath Statute was invalid where no special treatment facilities were available.[111]

Finding that offenders committed under the statute in fact were housed with other prisoners and received only such treatment as was available to the other prisoners, the court declared that commitment was in effect punishment and thus was in violation of the offenders' due process rights.[112] It is not enough, the court stated, for the legislature to announce a remedial purpose if the consequences to the individual in fact were penal.[113]

In 1966, the U.S. Court of Appeals for the District of Columbia held in *Millard v. Cameron* that indeterminate confinement under the District of Columbia's sexual psychopath law was justified only on a theory of therapeutic treatment.[114] The statute in question labeled committed offenders "patients"; thus, the court reasoned, the purpose of confinement must be to ensure treatment, not to exact retribution: "Lack of treatment destroys any otherwise valid reason for the differential consideration of the sexual psychopath."[115]

In 1982, the U.S. Court of Appeals for the Ninth Circuit, hearing a challenge to an Oregon law for committing sex offenders, ruled in *Ohlinger v. Watson* that mentally ill sex offenders committed for an indeterminate period of "treatment" have a constitutional right, under both the due process clause and the Eighth Amendment prohibition against cruel and unusual punishment, to such individual treatment as is necessary to provide a "realistic opportunity to be cured or to improve" their mental condition.[116] The court based its decision on the U.S. Supreme Court's opinion in *Jackson v. Indiana*.[117] In *Jackson*, the Supreme Court overturned the commitment of a man hospitalized for treatment to restore competency to stand trial on a criminal charge, noting that because the man (who was deaf and mute) was not treatable and therefore not likely to regain his competency in the "foreseeable future," his hospitalization served no legitimate purpose.[118] The nature and duration of a commitment must bear some "reasonable relation to the purpose for which the individual is committed," the Court declared.[119]

Although, *Jackson* aside, the U.S. Supreme Court has never clearly established that persons involuntarily committed to psychiatric hospitals have a right to treatment, the Court has addressed the issue at least peripherally in a number of cases. In *O'Connor v.*

Donaldson, decided in 1975, the Court held that it violated due process to involuntarily hospitalize, "without more," someone who could live safely in freedom.[120] Some scholars have suggested that the language "without more" was intended to refer to treatment—that commitment without treatment was unconstitutional, at least for persons who were not dangerous.[121] In *Youngberg v. Romeo,* decided in 1982, the Supreme Court held that a person with mental retardation who was confined in a state institution had a constitutional right to safe conditions of confinement and freedom from bodily restraint as well as such minimally adequate training as was required by these interests.[122] Although *Romeo* did not seek to enforce a right to treatment, per se, some commentators have interpreted this opinion to provide for a limited right to treatment.[123]

In *Allen v. Illinois,* decided in 1986, the U.S. Supreme Court ruled that Illinois' scheme for the hospitalization of "sexually dangerous persons" was civil and not criminal in nature because the law provided for *either* conviction and punishment *or* commitment and treatment for sexual psychopaths, not both.[124] The Court stated, "[i]n short, the State has disavowed any interest in punishment . . . , provided for the treatment of those it commits, and . . . established a system under which persons may be released after the briefest time in confinement."[125] This statement has been interpreted to suggest that the treatment provided as an alternative to punishment must have a possibility of success in order to be constitutional.[126]

Explanations and Solutions

The advent of determinate sentencing laws, restricting the authority of states to deny release to high-risk offenders, undoubtedly has much to do with the reemergence of sex offender commitment. Justice Wahl, in her dissenting opinion in *Blodgett,* observed that Minnesota's psychopathic personality statute, "infrequently invoked for many years, has come to be used increasingly to insure the detention of dangerous sex offenders *who have not been adequately controlled under determinate sentencing* [emphasis added]."[127] Justice

Wahl asked, "Why cannot the police power interest be vindicated by ordinary criminal processes, the use of enhanced sentences for recidivists, and other constitutionally permissible means?"[128]

Professor Peter Erlinger made this very point in his review of Washington's sexual predator law.[129] Erlinger concluded that the solution is not to create a new system of commitment but rather to impose longer sentences on all those convicted of sexual assault.[130] He argued that by prescribing life sentences for recidivists, the legislature could avoid the constitutional uncertainty surrounding its psychopathic personality statute, yet fulfill that statute's purpose: the detention of sexually dangerous persons.[131] Professor Brooks, however, in defense of the Washington State scheme, argued that sentencing all such offenders to life imprisonment would be overinclusive—that such a reform would have the effect of incapacitating many offenders who subsequently might prove to be good candidates for release.[132] One obvious solution, addressing the concerns of both Erlinger and Brooks, is simply to bring back indeterminate sentencing, at least for repeat sex offenders. By prescribing lengthy sentences (e.g., life) for certain categories of crime but allowing for discretionary parole, the state could ensure the retention of inmates deemed to be at high risk, yet allow for the release of lower-risk offenders, and it could do all this without the pretext of treatment. Treatment, of course, might be made available to offenders serving their sentences (and indeed, release decision making might turn, in some cases, on an offender's response to treatment), but pretending that treatment is the *purpose* of confinement would no longer be necessary.

References

1. Swanson AH: Sexual psychopath statutes: summary and analysis. 5 J Crim L & Criminology 215 (1960)
2. American Bar Association: Criminal justice mental health standards. Commentary to Standard 7–8.1, at 457 (1989) [hereinafter ABA Standards]
3. Brakel S, et al: The Mentally Disabled and the Law, 739. Chicago, IL, American Bar Foundation, 1985

4. Gleb G: Washington's sexually violent predator law: the need to bar unreliable psychiatric predictions of dangerousness from civil commitment proceedings. 39 UCLA L Rev 213, 215 (1991). Gleb states that Virginia was one of 13 states with sexual psychopath laws in 1990. Although Virginia had, and still has, a law providing for presentencing evaluations of sex offenders on court order, Virginia has never had a law for the special commitment of sex offenders. Thus, Gleb's count of 13 is reduced to 12 here.

5. Brakel et al, *supra* note 3, at 740

6. Fitch WL: States consider sex offender commitment laws. Networks, Spring 1998 (Published by National Technical Assistance Center for State Mental Health Planning, Alexandria, VA)

7. Minn Stat § 26.10 (1941). In upholding this law, the U.S. Supreme Court endorsed a Minnesota Supreme Court interpretation limiting the law's application to "those persons who, by an habitual course of misconduct in sexual matters, have evinced an utter lack of power to control their sexual impulses and . . . are likely to attack or otherwise inflict injury, loss, pain or other evil on the objects of their uncontrolled and uncontrollable desire." *Minnesota ex rel Pearson v Probate Court*, 309 US 270, 272 (1940). Despite this seemingly narrow reading, the law has been applied to Peeping Toms, self-abusers, and other nonviolent sexual "deviants." See, generally, cases that have permitted nonviolent sexual "deviants" to be committed as "sexual psychopaths": *In re Dittrich*, 215 Minn 234 (1943) (affirming a commitment on the basis of the respondent's "craving for sexual intercourse and self-abuse by masturbation," although he had never attacked or made any advances toward women); *State ex rel Haskett v Marion City Criminal Court*, 250 Ind 229 (1968) (defendant committed as a sexual psychopath after being charged with the crime of "peeping in a house"). *See also* Amy Kuebelbeck: Mental wards seen as drastic confinement for repeat rapists. Los Angeles Times, February 28, 1993, at A1 Col 1 ("In 1941, for example, men were committed for window-peeping, exposing themselves, masturbating and bestiality.").

8. Minn Stat § 253B.1(15) (1992)

9. Swanson, *supra* note 1, at 218. E.g., Ohio Rev Code Ann § 2947.25 (Baldwin 1958) ("After conviction and before sentence, a trial court must refer for examination all persons convicted under [special sections] of the Revised Code, to the department of mental hygiene and

correction or to a state facility designated by the department, or to a psychopathic clinic approved by the department. . . ."); Utah Code Ann § 77-49-1 (1953) ("Whenever any person is convicted of the offense of rape, sodomy, incest, lewdness, indecent exposure or carnal knowledge . . . the judge shall order a mental examination of such person. . . .").

10. *Id.* E.g., Ill Rev Stat Ch 38, § 822 (1959) ("When any person is charged with a criminal offense and it shall appear to the Attorney General or to the State's Attorney of the county wherein such person is so charged, that such person is a sexually dangerous person, then the Attorney General or State's Attorney . . . may file . . . a petition. . . . "); Wash Rev Code § 71.06.020 (1957) ("Where any person is charged in the superior court in this state with a sex offense and it appears that such person is a sexual psychopath, the prosecuting attorney may file a petition in the criminal proceeding, alleging that the defendant is a sexual psychopath and stating sufficient facts to support such allegation.").

11. *Id.*, at 216. E.g., Minn Stat § 526.10 (1975 & suppl 1992) ("The facts shall first be submitted to the county attorney, who, if he is satisfied that good cause exists, therefore, shall prepare the petition. . . ."); Neb Rev Stat § 29.2902 (suppl 1957) ("Whenever facts are presented to the county attorney which satisfy him that good cause exists for judicial inquiry . . . he shall prepare a petition. . . .").

12. *Id.* E.g., Ind Ann Stat § 9-3409 (suppl 1959) ("No person who is found . . . to be a criminal sexual psychopathic person . . . may thereafter be tried or sentenced upon the offense with which he originally stood charged or convicted. . . .").

13. *Id.*, at 219. E.g., Vt Stat Ann tit 18, § 2815 (1958) ("Upon his discharge from such confinement, such person shall be returned for sentence to the court wherein he was convicted.").

14. *Id. See* Ohio Rev Code Ann § 2947.27 (Baldwin 1958) ("If the person has been confined for a period less than the maximum sentence for the offense of which he was convicted, the order shall terminate the indefinite commitment. Thereupon the sentence which was suspended . . . shall forthwith go into effect and the person shall be transferred to the appropriate penal or reformatory institution. . . .").

15. La Fond JQ: Washington's sexually violent predator law: a deliberate misuse of the therapeutic state for social control. 15 U Puget

Sound L Rev 655, 661 (1992)

16. ABA Standards, *supra* note 2, at 457–8

17. Group for the Advancement of Psychiatry: Psychiatry and Sex Psychopath Legislation: The 30's to the 80's. New York, Group for the Advancement of Psychiatry, 1977 [hereinafter GAP Sex Psychopath Report]

18. ABA Standards, *supra* note 2, at 455

19. 4 Task Panel Reports, Submitted to the President's Commission on Mental Health 1978, at 1461 (1978)

20. GAP Sex Psychopath Report, *supra* note 17, at 935

21. *Id.*, at 843

22. Cross v Harris, 418 F2d 1095, 1107 (DC Cir 1969). Sexual psychopath laws have been challenged on procedural grounds as well. In Specht v Patterson, 386 US 605 (1967), the U.S. Supreme Court held that because persons charged as sexual psychopaths faced potentially indeterminate confinement, they had to be accorded certain fundamental legal protections, including the right to counsel, the right to a hearing, the right to present evidence, and the right to confront and cross-examine witnesses. In 1975, the U.S. Court of Appeals for the Seventh Circuit ruled that offenders could be committed under the Illinois Sexually Dangerous Persons Act only if found "beyond a reasonable doubt" to meet the standards for commitment. United States ex rel D v Coughlin 520 F2d 931 (7th Cir 1975).

23. ABA Standards, *supra* note 2, at 459. "Some legislatures came to feel that offenders were being released prematurely under such statutes, with consequent danger to public safety."

24. Ransley MT: Note, Repeal of the Wisconsin Sex Crimes Act. 1980 Wis L Rev 941, 953 (1980)

25. *Id.*

26. *Id.*, at 951–953

27. Gleb, *supra* note 4. In 1990, 12 states and the District of Columbia had sexual psychopath statutes: Colorado, Connecticut, the District of Columbia, Illinois, Massachusetts, Minnesota, Nebraska, New Jersey, Oregon, Tennessee, Utah, and Washington.

28. *See* Von Hirsch A: Doing Justice: The Choice of Punishments. Boston, MA, Northeastern University Press, 1986

29. *See* Allen FA: Criminal justice, legal values, and the rehabilitative ideal. 50 J Crim L Criminology, and Police Science 226 (1959), dis-

cussed in La Fond, *supra* note 15, at 664

30. La Fond, *supra* note 15, at 664
31. Von Hirsch A, Haurahan P: Determinate penalty systems in America: an overview. 27 Crime Delinq 289 (1981)
32. Tonry MH: Real offense sentencing: the Model Sentencing and Correction Act. 72 J Crim L Criminology 1550, 1551 (1981)
33. *Id.*
34. *Id.* In many states, however, the prescribed penalty may be adjusted to some degree based on a finding of particular aggravating or mitigating circumstances.
35. Wash Laws Ch 137
36. "Presumptive" sentences are calculated primarily on the basis of the offense of conviction and the nature and extent of the offender's criminal record. The actual sentence may be adjusted slightly to account for particular mitigating or aggravating circumstances.
37. Wash Rev Code § 9.94 A. 310–320 (suppl 1990–1991)
38. Wash Rev Code § 71.09.010 (suppl 1990–1991)
39. Gleb, *supra* note 4, at 213–214. *See also* Boerner D: Confronting violence: in the act and in the world. 15 Puget Sound L Rev 525 (1992)
40. *Id.*
41. *Id.*
42. *Id.*
43. La Fond, *supra* note 15, at 655
44. Wash Rev Code § 71.09.010 (West 1975 & suppl 1991)
45. La Fond, *supra* note 15, at 656
46. *Id.*
47. Wash Rev Code Ann § 71.09.030 (suppl 1990–1991)
48. Wash Stat Ann § 71.09.020(2) (West 1975 & suppl 1990)
49. Wash Rev Code Ann § 71.09.030 (West 1975 & suppl 1991). *See also* Bochnewich MA: Comment, prediction of dangerousness and Washington's sexually violent predator statute. 29 Cal W L Rev 277 (1992)
50. Wash Rev Code Ann § 71.09.40 (West 1975 & suppl 1991)
51. *Id.*
52. *In re* Young, 857 P2d 989, 993 (Wash 1993)
53. *Id.*
54. Wash Rev Code Ann § 71.09.050 (West 1975 & suppl 1991). "The person, the prosecuting attorney or attorney general, or the judge shall have the right to demand that the trial be before a jury. If no

demand is made, the trial shall be before the court."

55. Wash Rev Code Ann § 71.09.060 (West 1975 & suppl 1991)
56. Gleb, *supra* note 4, at 216
57. Wash Rev Code Ann § 71.09.060(1) (West 1975 & suppl 1991)
58. Telephone interview with Terry Davis, Director of Quality Enhancement, Kansas Department of Mental Health (June 22, 1994)
59. Anderson NW, Masters KW: Predators and politics: the dichotomies of translation in the Washington sexually violent predators statute. 15 U Puget Sound L Rev 507 (1992)
60. 857 P2d 989 (Wash 1993)
61. Young v Weston, 898 F Supp 744 (WD Wash 1995)
62. The double jeopardy clause prohibits multiple punishments for the same offense. United States v Halper, 449 US 435, 448 (1989). The ex post facto prohibition is aimed at laws that allow for greater punishment than was possible when the crime was committed or make it more difficult for the defense at trial than would have been the case at the time of the crime. Calder v Bull, 3 US 386 (1798).
63. *In re* Young, 857 P2d 998 (Wash 1993)64.
64. *In re Young*, at 1003
65. *In re Young*, at 1005
66. Brooks AD: The constitutionality and morality of civilly committing violent sexual predators. 15 U Puget Sound L Rev 709, 733 (1992)
67. *In re Young*, at 1001
68. *Id.*, at 1002
69. *Id.*
70. Wash Rev Code § 71.09.010 (suppl 1990–1991)
71. *Id.*
72. *In re Young*, at 1003
73. *Id.*
74. Wash Rev Code § 71.05.020 (3) (West 1975 & suppl 1991)
75. *In re Young*, at 1009
76. *Id.*, at 1011, quoting Baxstrom v Herold, 383 US 107, 111 (1966)
77. *Id.*, at 1010
78. *Id.*
79. *Id.*, at 1014
80. *Id.*, at 1012
81. *Id.*, at 1021
82. *Id.*, at 1020
83. *Id.*, at 1022

84. *Id.*, at 1019
85. Young v Weston, 898 F Supp 744 (1995)
86. Foucha v Louisiana, 112 S Ct 1787 (1991)
87. State v Post and State v Oldakowski, 197 Wis 2d 279 (December 1995)
88. *Id.*, at 14
89. *Id.*, at 19
90. O'Connor v Donaldson, 422 US 563, 589 (1975)
91. *Post, Oldakowski*, at 19
92. *Id.*, at dissent 19
93. Minnesota *ex rel* Pearson v Probate Court of Ramsey County Minn 309 US 270 (1940)
94. *In re* Blodgett, 510 NW2d 910 (1994)
95. *Id.*
96. *In re* Blodgett, 490 NW2d 638 (Minn App 1992)
97. *In re* Blodgett, 510 NW2d 910, 914 (1994). In *Foucha,* the U.S. Supreme Court held that it violates the Constitution to confine in a psychiatric hospital a person acquitted of a criminal offense by reason of insanity who was no longer mentally ill. In dicta, the Court observed that the state may confine under its police power 1) convicted criminals (for the purpose of deterrence and retribution); 2) persons mentally ill and dangerous; and 3) for a limited time under "certain narrow circumstances [i.e., while awaiting trial on serious criminal charges] persons who pose a danger to others or to the community." Foucha v Louisiana, 112 S Ct 1780, 1785–1786 (1992).
98. *Id.*
99. *Id.*
100. *Id.*, at 916
101. *Id.*, at 912
102. *Id.*, at 916
103. *Id.*
104. *Id.*, at 918
105. *Id.*
106. *Id.*, at 925
107. *Id.*
108. Kansas v Hendricks, 117 S Ct 2072 (1997)
109. "For purposes of my argument in this dissent . . . the material that the majority wishes to consider, when read in its entirety, shows that Kansas was not providing treatment to Hendricks."

110. Fitch WL: Sex offender commitment in the United States. Journal of Forensic Psychiatry 9(2):240, 1998

111. Commonwealth v Page, 159 NE2d 82 (Mass 1959)

112. *Id.*, at 317–318

113. *Id.*

114. Millard v Cameron, 373 F2d 478 (DC Cir 1966)

115. *Id.*, at 473

116. Ohlinger v Watson, 652 F2d 775, 777 (9th Cir 1980)

117. Jackson v Indiana, 406 US 715 (1971)

118. *Id.*

119. *Id.*

120. O'Connor v Donaldson, 422 US 563 (1975)

121. *See,* for example, Gutheil TG, Applebaum PS: Clinical Handbook of Psychiatry and the Law. New York, McGraw-Hill, 1982, at 82

122. Youngberg v Romeo, 475 US 307 (1982)

123. La Fond JQ: Washington's sexually violent predators statute: law or lottery? A response to Professor Brooks. 15 U Puget Sound L Rev 755, 766 (1992)

124. Allen v Illinois, 478 US 364 (1986)

125. *Id.*, at 370

126. La Fond, *supra* note 123, at 767

127. *In re Blodgett,* 510 NW2d at 920

128. *Id.*, at 924

129. Erlinger P: Minnesota's Gulag: involuntary treatment for the "politically ill." 19 William Mitchell L Rev 99 (1993)

130. *Id.*

131. *Id.*

132. Brooks, *supra* note 76, at 752

CHAPTER 3

Paraphilias: Prevalence, Characteristics, Evaluation, and Cognitive-Behavior Treatment

Introduction

Paraphilic Interests in the Nonclinical Population

It is difficult to determine the frequency of paraphilic interests in nonclinical populations because it is problematic to obtain representative samples of the general population, especially when sensitive issues such as sexuality are being examined, and because individuals are reluctant to report sexual interests that may be divergent from those of the general population. Crepault and Coulture[1] questioned 94 men regarding their sexual fantasies during masturbation or intercourse. Of this population, 61.7% reported fantasies of initiating a young girl into sexuality; 33.0% described fantasies of raping adult women; 11.7% described masochistic fantasies; 5.3% described fantasies of having sex with an animal; and 3.2% described fantasies of initiating a young boy into sexuality. Templeman and Stinnett[2] investigated 60 male undergraduate college students regarding their participation in and/or fantasies of paraphilic behavior. Of these students, 42% reported having participated in voyeurism; 35%, in frottage; 8%, in making obscene telephone calls; 5%, in coercive sexual activity; 3%, in sexual contact with girls under age 12; and 2%, in exhibitionism. A total of 65% reported having participated in some variant of paraphilic behavior. In this same population, 54% reported a desire to be involved in voyeuristic behavior; 7% reported a desire to participate in exhibitionistic behavior; and 5% reported a desire to be sexual with girls under age 12.

Examining these nonclinical populations suggests that paraphilic interests are fairly common in men and include a wide variety of paraphilic interests or behaviors typically seen in clinical populations seeking evaluation and treatment for paraphilias.

Characteristics of Individuals Seeking Evaluation and Treatment for Possible Paraphilias

Individuals seeking evaluation and treatment in the clinical setting are unlikely to be representative samples of persons with paraphilias. Some paraphilic behaviors, such as the use of fetish objects, usually take place in private and thus do not come to the attention of others unless they are revealed by the paraphilic person. Other categories of paraphilic behavior (such as voyeurism and exhibitionism) may occur frequently, but because of the transient nature of the act and the lack of a relationship between the participants, these behaviors infrequently lead to arrests and therefore come to the attention of health care providers only when they become habitual or lead to social consequences for the paraphilic person. Some paraphilias are overrepresented in psychiatric facilities because they frequently lead to identification of the perpetrator. Mandatory reporting laws for child molestation and incest, as well as public outrage over the rape of adults, increase the likelihood that individuals accused of aggressive sexual behavior will come to the attention of psychiatric facilities.

Recent data gathered from more than 90 treatment programs throughout North America regarding 2,129 cases of individuals seeking assessment (see Figure 1–1) indicate that 37.1% had been involved in child molestation; 20.2%, in voyeurism; 13.8%, in exhibitionism; 13.3%, in fetishism; 11.2%, in frottage; and 10.7%, in public masturbation. The remaining categories of paraphilia were reported at lower frequencies. Psychiatrists wishing to evaluate and treat patients with paraphilias should be especially acquainted with the paraphilias most likely to be encountered in evaluation or treatment facilities.

A study of 561 paraphilic persons[3] who had committed more than 291,000 paraphilic acts against more than 195,000 victims indicated that, of all victims, 37.3% were victims of exhibitionism; 28.6%, of frottage; 13.6%, of voyeurism; 11.8%, of molestation against boys outside the home; 3.5%, of public masturbation; 2.3%, of molestation of girls outside the home; 1%, of obscene telephone calls; 0.9%, of bestiality; 0.5%, of rape of adult women; 0.2%, of molestation of girls in the home; 0.2%, of urolagnia; and 0.1% or less, of sadism, masochism, fetishism, molestation of boys within the home, obscene mailings, coprophilia, or attraction to odors. These results suggest that most victims of paraphilic acts are victims of exhibitionism, frottage, voyeurism, and molestation of boys outside the home.

The frequency with which persons with paraphilias carry out paraphilic behavior shows marked variance. This frequency extends from individuals who only have the urges to commit the acts but have never actually done so to paraphilic persons who have committed thousands of acts during their lifetime. The average number of acts per paraphilic person is unlikely to be representative of what paraphilic persons actually do, because in each category of paraphilia there are some persons who commit acts at an exceedingly high frequency and thereby markedly exaggerate the average number of acts committed in each category of paraphilia. For this reason, the median is a better representation of the frequency of acts by paraphilic persons.

In the sample mentioned earlier,[3] the median numbers of paraphilic acts by paraphilic category are as follows: nonincestuous molestation of a female victim, 1.4; nonincestuous molestation of a male victim, 10.1; incestuous molestation of a female victim, 4.4; incestuous molestation of a male victim, 5.2; rape of adult women, 0.9; exhibitionism, 50.5; voyeurism, 16.5; frottage, 29.5; transvestism, 25.0; fetishism, 3.3; sadism, 3.0; masochism,

36.0; obscene telephone calls, 30.0; public masturbation, 50.0; and bestiality, 2.2. Clearly, despite a low frequency of arrest, the median number of paraphilic acts is high, as in cases of exhibitionism, voyeurism, frottage, transvestism, masochism, obscene telephone calls, and public masturbation. Masochistic acts, specifically, occur at a high frequency because generally they are done with only a few consistent partners.

Fortunately, when the paraphilic behavior involves touching of the victim, the use of force, or nonconsenting victims (such as rape or child molestation), the median number of paraphilic acts is low. Of the latter category of paraphilic behaviors, molestation of boys outside the home has the highest median number of acts.

Early studies of paraphilic persons suggested that such persons usually become compulsively involved with a single category of paraphilic behavior and infrequently cross over into other categories of paraphilia. A more recent study[4] suggests that this is not the case. Of paraphilic persons primarily involved with actual touching of their victims (e.g., frottage, rape, and pedophilia), 30.6% had previously or concomitantly been involved in paraphilic acts not involving touching of the victim (e.g., voyeurism and exhibitionism). Of paraphilic persons primarily involved with hands-off paraphilic acts against their victims, 64.0% had previously or concomitantly carried out paraphilic acts involving actual touching of the victim. Of paraphilic persons primarily victimizing individuals outside the family, 29.4% had previously or concomitantly carried out paraphilic acts against family members. Of those who primarily had been involved in paraphilic acts with family members, 65.8% had previously or concomitantly carried out paraphilic sexual acts against non–family members. Of paraphilic persons who primarily committed acts against female victims, 22.9% had previously or concomitantly carried out paraphilic acts against male victims. Of those who had primarily carried out paraphilic acts against male victims, 62.6% had previously or concomitantly carried out paraphilic acts against female victims as well.

Of those who had targeted victims age 13 or younger, 43% had previously or concomitantly been involved in paraphilic acts against adolescent victims, and 34.4% against adult victims. Of those who had targeted victims ages 14–17, 67.3% had previously or concomitantly committed paraphilic acts against children age 13 or younger, and 42.6% against victims age 18 years or older. Of those who had committed paraphilic acts against adults, 49.2% had previously or concomitantly committed paraphilic acts against children age 13 or younger, and 38.9% against adolescents ages 14–17.

This information indicates that paraphilic persons tend to cross over between touching and nontouching of their victims, between family and non–family members, between female and male victims, and to victims of various ages.

Table 3–1[4a] demonstrates the same crossing-over process in terms of selection of the paraphilic acts committed. In a study of 859 paraphilic persons, each was categorized according to the most prominent paraphilic behavior (the primary diagnosis), as well as other, less prominent paraphilic behaviors in which he or she was previously or concomitantly involved (secondary diagnosis). To determine the secondary diagnoses associated with a particular primary diagnosis, locate the horizontal row containing the primary diagnosis and the vertical column containing the secondary diagnosis. For example, of paraphilic persons whose primary diagnosis was male nonincest pedophilia, 120 such individuals were seen. Of these, 37% were previously or concomitantly involved with female nonincest pedophilia; 5%, with female incest pedophilia; 13%, with male incest pedophilia; 3%, with rape of adult women; 12%, with exhibitionism; 10%, with voyeurism; 5%, with frottage; 2%, with obscene mail; 0%, with transsexualism; 4%, with transvestism; 2%, with fetishism; 5%, with sadism; 3%, with masochism; 0%, with ego-dystonic homosexuality; 0%, with obscene telephone calling; 1%, with public masturbation; 3%, with bestiality; 1%, with urolagnia; 0%, with coprophilia; and 0%, with arousal to specific odors. (Categories having fewer than 10 subjects were excluded because they were believed not to be adequately represented.) Examining other primary diagnostic paraphilic categories leads to the conclusion that crossing into other categories of paraphilia is common.

The criteria for determining which paraphilia is the most prob-

Table 3–1. Cross-diagnosis by paraphilia

Secondary diagnosis

Primary diagnosis	Female nonincest pedophilia	Male nonincest pedophilia	Female incest pedophilia	Male incest pedophilia	Rape	Exhibitionism	Voyeurism	Frottage	Obscene mail
Female nonincest pedophilia	100	22	30	7	10	18	14	7	0
Male nonincest pedophilia	37	100	5	13	3	12	10	5	2
Female incest pedophilia	19	5	100	6	10	10	7	3	1
Male incest pedophilia	27	32	32	100	18	6	18	9	3
Rape	17	2	5	0	100	11	14	6	1
Exhibitionism	13	8	12	3	14	100	27	17	0
Voyeurism	15	0	4	0	33	26	100	11	0
Frottage	14	0	1	0	14	17	14	100	0
Obscene mail	0	0	0	0	0	0	0	0	100
Transsexualism	0	0	0	0	0	0	0	0	0
Transvestism	5	5	0	0	0	5	15	0	5
Fetishism	17	8	8	8	8	8	8	8	8
Sadism	36	18	18	0	46	9	36	9	0
Masochism	8	0	0	0	15	15	23	8	0
Ego-dystonic homosexuality	4	4	0	7	0	7	0	0	4
Obscene phone calling	0	0	13	0	13	13	25	0	0
Public masturbation	18	6	12	0	12	29	41	12	0
Bestiality	33	17	17	17	0	0	50	0	0
Urolagnia	0	0	0	0	0	0	0	0	0
Coprophilia	0	0	0	0	0	0	0	0	0
Arousal to odors	0	0	0	0	0	0	0	0	0

Note. Numbers are percentages.

Secondary diagnosis

Transsexualism	Transvestism	Fetishism	Sadism	Masochism	Ego-dystonic homosexuality	Obscene phone calling	Public masturbation	Bestiality	Urolagnia	Coprophilia	Arousal to odors
0	2	5	1	2	1	5	2	7	1	1	1
0	4	2	5	3	0	0	1	3	1	0	0
1	5	3	3	1	1	1	1	4	1	1	0
0	3	12	3	0	0	3	3	9	0	3	0
0	2	1	9	0	0	5	4	4	0	0	1
1	5	4	3	3	1	3	10	4	1	0	0
0	7	15	0	4	0	7	7	11	0	0	0
0	0	11	8	0	3	6	0	6	0	0	3
0	0	0	0	50	0	0	0	0	0	0	0
100	7	0	0	0	15	0	0	0	0	0	0
15	100	20	0	1	15	5	5	10	0	0	0
0	33	100	17	33	0	0	17	0	0	0	0
0	9	0	100	9	0	0	0	0	0	0	0
0	15	8	23	100	8	0	0	23	15	0	0
19	22	7	0	0	100	0	0	4	4	0	0
0	25	25	0	13	0	100	13	25	13	0	0
0	6	18	12	0	0	6	100	12	1	0	0
0	33	33	0	33	17	33	0	100	17	17	17
0	0	0	0	0	0	0	0	0	0	0	0
0	0	0	0	0	0	0	0	0	0	0	0
0	0	0	0	0	0	0	0	0	0	0	0

lematic could include the number of victims, the number of acts completed, the degree of aggressiveness, or any number of other factors. One possible criterion might be the likelihood of crossing into other categories of paraphilia, suggesting a lack of discrimination in paraphilic acts. This tendency to cross into other diagnostic categories can be tabulated from Table 3–1 by adding the percentage of individuals with each primary diagnosis to the percentage of those who also cross into other secondary paraphilic diagnoses.

Using this criterion of crossing into other secondary paraphilic acts, the paraphilias with the highest incidence of crossover were, in decreasing order, sadism, public masturbation, male incest pedophilia, fetishism, masochism, voyeurism, female nonincest pedophilia, exhibitionism, male nonincest pedophilia, transvestism, frottage, female incest pedophilia, rape of adult women, ego-dystonic homosexuality, and transsexualism.

Probably the most impressive aspects of Table 3–1 and the crossing of diagnoses are the categories of paraphilias in which crossing is limited—that is, transsexualism, ego-dystonic homosexuality, rape of adult females, and female incest pedophilia. It is not surprising that transsexualism and ego-dystonic homosexuality have low crossing of diagnosis, since DSM-IV does not consider them to be paraphilias. The fact that rape of adult females has such a low crossing of diagnosis suggests that rapists of adult females, at least those who seek psychiatric care, may not actually have a paraphilia. Female incest pedophilia, likewise, may be more the result of the availability of the female child family member than a recurrent, compulsive paraphilic interest.

Assessment of Persons With a Paraphilia

Clinical Interview

Clinical interviews with persons who may have a paraphilia should begin with obtaining the patient's written, voluntary informed consent for the assessment (or the consent of the patient's guardian), even if the assessment is court-ordered. The consent form should identify the components of the assessment protocol, the risks and benefits of the assessment, the patient's right to refuse the assessment, the limits of confidentiality, child abuse reporting requirements, and what to do if the patient experiences any problems as a result of the assessment procedure. The patient's signature should be witnessed after all his questions regarding consent have been answered. When interviewing adolescents or other patients who have a guardian, it is advisable to get not only the guardian's consent but also the patient's signature as well. Guardians should be offered the opportunity to view all assessment materials before giving their consent for the assessment. A written statement should verify that the guardian was given this opportunity and either viewed or did not view these materials.

Interviewing techniques with persons who may have a paraphilia should be based on the supposition that the patient has carried out a paraphilic act and will discuss it with the interviewer. It is also imperative that the interviewer avoid allowing the patient to voice denial of paraphilic acts early in the interview, because once such a denial has been expressed it will be difficult for the patient to later admit his actions. Questions such as "Have you committed any sex crimes?" suggest to the patient that denial is an option for him. Questions should instead focus on the expectation of reporting paraphilic acts, such as "How long have you been sexually involved with children?"

It is also important to avoid the offender's use of labels; that is, the clinician should be interested in the person's behavior, not in how the person might label it. Terms such as *molest* are too vague because they encompass a wide variety of behaviors. The interviewer should obtain detailed information about the specific acts the person has carried out, the duration of the behavior, the first occurrence of the behavior, any possible antecedents that trigger the person's deviant interests, and the frequency of the behavior.

One common interviewer error is not questioning the patient about all types of paraphilias. As Table 3–1 illustrates, many individuals coming for treatment have more than one paraphilia or have carried out more than one type of paraphilic act. If not specifically asked about various paraphilic interests, many patients will not volunteer this information. Most offenders only report behaviors that have come to the attention of others. It is advisable to have a list of the various paraphilias and to go through the list, questioning the patient about each type of paraphilia. In this way, the interviewer is more likely to identify the full extent of the patient's paraphilic interests so that they may all be addressed in therapy. It is also helpful at this point to question the patient about possible sexual dysfunctions.

When the patient denies any paraphilic interests or behaviors, the interviewer should focus on what others have said he did—for example, what he has been charged with or what is in the victim's statement. Once this information is established, the interviewer should avoid asking questions that challenge what the patient says. Rather, the interviewer should ask for clarification about the incident, the patient's relationship with the alleged victim, and other relevant factors. If the patient continues to deny any involvement whatsoever in the reported paraphilic behavior, the interviewer should not schedule numerous appointments in an attempt to establish a "relationship" with the patient in the hope that the patient will eventually admit his behavior. This is a time-consuming and generally unproductive approach. It also allows significant time to pass without the patient receiving treatment, potentially placing additional individuals at risk for victimization. A quicker, more efficient way to break through the patient's denial is through the use of psychophysiological measures such as plethysmography, visual reaction time, and/or polygraphy, which are discussed below.

Psychological Assessment

Standard psychological tests (such as intelligence tests, projective and objective personality tests, and neuropsychological tests) are not particularly helpful with persons alleged to have a paraphilia because these instruments are designed to assess such factors as intelligence and personality types—factors that do not differentially identify paraphilia. These tests can help to determine the psychological profile of a given offender and thus may be useful to the treating clinician, but there is no evidence at present that they can be validly used to determine whether an individual has paraphilia.[1,2]

Some psychological tests address issues that are relevant to understanding and treating paraphilic persons. These tests rely on the self-report of the person being tested but can help to identify inappropriate sexual interests or issues relevant to treatment, such as social inadequacy, cognitive distortions, alcoholism, and personality disorders. Many of these instruments can also be used to measure treatment progress (pre-post measures). Some of the most frequently used tests are the 1) Abel and Becker Cognition Scale, 2) Attitudes Toward Women Scale, 3) Burt Rape Myth Acceptance Scale, 4) Buss-Durkee Hostility Inventory, 5) Hare Psychopathy Scale, 6) Multiphasic Sex Inventory, 7) Abel and Becker Sexual Interest Card Sort, 8) Clarke Sexual History Questionnaire, 9) Interpersonal Reactivity Index, 10) Minnesota Multiphasic Personality Inventory, 11) Family Adaptability and Cohesion Evaluation Scale, 12) Social Avoidance and Distress Scale, 13) Mosher Forced-Choice Inventory, 14) Michigan Alcohol Screening Test, and 15) Millon Clinical Multiaxial Inventory.[5,6]

Psychophysiological Assessment

The primary feature that separates individuals with paraphilia from those who do not have paraphilia is their specific sexual attraction to unusual behavior, nonhuman objects, or sexual activities involving nonconsent. Since paraphilic persons are prone to conceal their true arousal pattern, it is not surprising that assessment methods have been developed that do not rely on admission of paraphilic interests.

Plethysmography. In 1971, Zuckerman[7] reviewed various physiological means for identifying sexual interest and found that direct measurement of sexual response was the most effective. Penile plethysmography, initially described by Freund,[8] involves measuring volume changes in the penis or circumferential measures of the penis while concomitantly presenting the patient with stimuli involving discrete categories of paraphilic stimuli. These stimuli might be presented as slides, audiotaped descriptions, or videos depicting the categories to be investigated. A person suspected of pedophilia, for example, will undergo plethysmographic measurement while viewing slides depicting males or females of various ages, thus producing a generalization gradient reflecting the degree of sexual arousal to males and/or females of various ages. Persons suspected of sadism will be shown depictions of sadomasochistic acts; those suspected of voyeurism, slides photographed through a window depicting women undressing; and those suspected of fetishism, various fetish objects. Murphy and Barbaree[9] and others have reviewed the uses of penile plethysmography and its advantages and disadvantages. Initially plethysmography was used with "admitters"—individuals who admitted to their paraphilic interest. In more recent years, laboratories have investigated arousal patterns of noncompliant, nonadmitting possible paraphilic persons. As a result, the various factors that might inhibit the validity of plethysmographic measurements have become more and more important. Therapists who use plethysmography as an essential component of assessment—to evaluate the treatment needs and response to treatment of persons with a paraphilia—have carried such measurements into the courtroom. The courtroom has unfortunately become an arena for the discussion of variables affecting the validity of plethysmography.

Factors that can have an impact on the validity of such measures include

1. *Not attending to the stimuli.* Some paraphilic persons attempt concealment of their paraphilic interests by avoiding looking at or listening to the depictions of paraphilic acts. Measures to counteract this tendency include asking the person to describe the stimuli presented, asking the person to identify signals superimposed on the stimuli (signal detection), and directly observing the person's visual gaze during assessment.

2. *Voluntary suppression.* Despite attending to the stimuli, some individuals can suppress their responsiveness by imagining other stimuli or carrying out distracting mental tasks.[10] Coun-

termeasures have included having the patient verbalize an encounter with the person in the stimulus being viewed, or instructing the individual at times to suppress and at other times not to suppress their arousal, in order to establish the person's baseline ability to suppress arousal intentionally. Still others ignore this issue and instead view the individual's ability to suppress arousal in the laboratory as good evidence that therapy has been effective, in that the individual has learned to control his arousal.

3. *Normative data.* A major problem with such testing has been the sensitivity, specificity, and efficiency of the testing procedure. In testing persons suspected of pedophilia using both the volumetric and circumferential penile plethysmography devices, these factors have been established. For volumetric phallometry, the sensitivity is 87, the specificity is 95, and the efficiency is 95. With the circumferential device, the sensitivity is 48, the specificity is 100, and the efficiency is 97 (Table 3–2).[11] The sensitivities of these testing methods for persons suspected of raping adult women have yet to be determined, and there is considerable disagreement in the literature regarding the effectiveness of plethysmography with those suspected of raping adult females. Virtually no sensitivity, specificity, or efficiency data are available on plethysmography with other paraphilias.

4. *Lack of standardized stimuli.* A further problem with plethysmography is that the stimuli presented during testing have not been standardized. Initially, the National Institute of Mental Health (NIMH) and some of the major sex offender evaluation and treatment programs in North America attempted to arrive at a standard set of stimuli for use with those suspected of pedophilia that involved males and females ages 4, 8, 12, 16, and 24. Although a number of states in the United States allow the use of depictions of children for scientific or medical purposes, federal law is likely to consider the transport across state lines of stimuli depicting nude children as a federal offense. In 1993, concerns were voiced nationwide that therapists using such stimuli could be arrested, and this threat of arrest has had a profound damping effect on the use of such stimuli. The ab-

Table 3–2.   Sensitivity, specificity, and efficiency of tests assuming 5% prevalence of the disorder

Test/disorder	Sensitivity (%)	Specificity (%)	Efficiency (%)
Urine test for diabetes mellitus	44	97	94
Blood test for diabetes mellitus	64	97	95
ECG for left ventricular enlargement	58	97	95
MAST for alcoholism	100	70	71
Volumetric plethysmography for pedophilia	87	95	95
Circumferential plethysmography for pedophilia	48	100	97
Abel screen for risk of behavior			
With prepubescent boys	76	98	97
With pubescent boys	90	98	98
With prepubescent girls	91	77	78
With pubescent girls	86	77	78

Note.   Adapted from Ref. 11. ECG = electrocardiogram; MAST = Michigan Alcohol Screening Test.

sence of standardized stimuli has further scientific repercussions in that if data are to be compared from one treatment program to another, identical stimuli need to be used. The United States federal law conflicts with the scientific needs of those evaluating and treating persons with paraphilias, and this issue remains unresolved.

5. *Denial of paraphilic interest.* One way of dealing with the lack of standardization is to confront the person with the results of his own psychophysiological measurement[12] (as opposed to comparing the individual's responses to paraphilic and "normal" stimuli with the responses of either nonparaphilic persons or other persons with paraphilias). Some individuals being as-

sessed for possible paraphilic interest will flatly deny having any such interest either historically or at the time of plethysmographic measurement. In such circumstances, when arousal to deviant stimuli is measured and the person is confronted with the inconsistency of measured versus reported paraphilic interests, 62% of persons suspected of having a paraphilia report paraphilic interest that they had previously denied. As a result, the number of diagnoses of paraphilia is doubled.

This confrontation methodology appears to be effective, in part because persons who come for assessment for possible paraphilias never reveal that they have paraphilic arousal (that could be measured physiologically) but simply do not act on it. Instead, they deny any paraphilic interest whatsoever and usually say the same in the laboratory. As a consequence, when erection responses to paraphilic stimuli are recorded, these responses contradict the person's prior denial.

6. *Variation, duration, and quantity of erection measurement.* Plethysmography involves the presentations of paraphilic and nonparaphilic stimuli, the durations of which vary greatly from one laboratory to another. As a result, the outcome of assessments varies. A further source of variance is the manner in which erection response is measured. In the United States, all measures are made using the circumferential penile transducer, identical to that used during nocturnal penile tumescence monitoring in the discrimination of rapid-eye-movement (REM) versus non-REM sleep, or differential diagnosis of organic versus psychogenic erectile dysfunction. In some laboratories in Canada, measures are obtained by the volumetric device described by Freund[8,13]—a glass casing enclosing the penis up to the base—which quantifies the gas displacement resulting from an erection during stimulus presentation. The volumetric device measures minute (sometimes less than 1 mm^3) changes in penile volume, whereas circumferential measures traditionally depend on the patient getting at least 10% of an erection before the data can be used. The consequence of these differences is that the volumetric device can measure small

changes, whereas the circumferential device necessitates significant response on the patient's part. Because most men can sense at least 20% of an erection, circumferential measures are potentially subject to voluntary control by the subject, because he can detect his erection response to some of the stimuli. With the volumetric device this is less of a problem, and therefore volumetric device measurements have greater validity.

7. *The relationship between plethysmography in the laboratory and the patient's behavior outside the laboratory.* Murphy and Barbaree[9] have attempted to clarify that laboratory responses cannot be used to predict or validate behaviors outside the laboratory. Each of us, at times, has arousal that, if we acted on it, could be quite problematic. Having arousal, be it paraphilic or non-paraphilic, does not mean that we necessarily act on that arousal. Plethysmography results are frequently used inappropriately in making judgments regarding the veracity of an individual's claim that he did or did not participate in paraphilic behavior outside of the laboratory. However, irrespective of the desires of plaintiffs and defendants in such cases, plethysmography cannot provide definitive answers to such complex questions. As a result, it is considered inappropriate to use plethysmography measures to argue the issue of the veracity of an individual's statement regarding previous behavior. Notwithstanding the inappropriate attempts to use plethysmography in the courtroom, plethysmography is exceedingly valuable in the therapy setting, since it is one of the most cost-effective means of confronting denial and measuring the person's response to therapy.

Visual reaction time. A more recent means of assessing sexual interest is called visual reaction time, visual fixation time, or viewing time. Use of the visual reaction time methodology was initially reported in the early 1940s for measuring individuals' adult sexual preferences.[14] A number of authors[11,15–20] have refined this methodology to objectively measure adult sexual preference and, more recently, to measure an individual's sexual interest in males or females ages 2–4, 8–10, and 14–17 and in male or female adults.[11,21]

In general, the individual being assessed uses a computer to advance slides depicting individuals of various ages, sexes, and ethnicity. The computer measures the amount of time the individual spends looking at each category of stimuli and also records the individual's self-reported sexual arousal to each slide.

Visual reaction time testing has a number of advantages over other means of assessment, including the following:

1. There is a relatively brief administration time (the entire assessment takes less than an hour to complete);
2. No special laboratory is needed;
3. It can be used with males or females of any age down to age 12 years;
4. The sexual interest measurements can be made with depictions of nonnude stimuli.

Visual reaction time testing has recently been compared with penile plethysmography[21] and has been found to have similar reliability and validity to penile plethysmography. As with penile plethysmography, it has its highest sensitivity and specificity when measuring an individual's possible sexual interest in adolescent or prepubescent boys, with less sensitivity and specificity when measuring possible sexual interest in adolescent or prepubescent girls. Its high sensitivity and specificity suggest that it may be used to screen out individuals with sexual interest in children who are applying to work in youth organizations.

Visual reaction time testing, like plethysmography, includes some factors that may affect its validity, including

1. *Not attending to the stimuli.* Because the visual reaction time method involves measurement of the time the individual spends looking at the stimuli, the patient's attempts to look elsewhere are generally reduced by asking the individual to carry out a task necessitating his or her attending to the stimuli, such as self-reporting sexual interest to the slide, or completing a signal detection task while looking at each slide.
2. *Voluntary suppression.* Studies have examined the ease with

which individuals can falsify visual reaction times. Results show that although absolute visual reaction times can be suppressed, the relative suppression of visual reaction time remains unchanged, so that the relative sexual interest that individuals might demonstrate on visual reaction time tests holds constant, whether they are asked to undergo the assessment honestly or to falsify the task so as to appear perfectly normal.

3. *Normative data.* The ease of measuring visual reaction time has allowed the sensitivity, specificity, and efficiency of the testing procedure to be determined with subcategories of sexual interest in children. Measurement with prepubescent male stimuli gives a sensitivity of 76%, a specificity of 98%, and an efficiency of 96.9%. Identifying sexual interest in pubescent boys yields a sensitivity of 90%, a specificity of 98%, and an efficiency of 97.6%. Identifying those with interest in prepubescent girls yields a sensitivity of 91%, a specificity of 77%, and an efficiency of 77.7%. Identifying those with sexual interest in pubescent girls yields a sensitivity of 86%, a specificity of 77%, and an efficiency of 77.5%.

Currently, visual reaction time assessment is used primarily to examine an individual's relative sexual interest in persons of various age and gender categories.

4. *Lack of standardized stimuli.* To date there is no standard set of stimuli used for visual reaction time assessment. However, because visual reaction time testing does not require nude depictions of children as stimuli, it is possible to transport stimuli of nonnude children across state lines, and therefore there is no obstruction to the distribution of a standard set of stimuli.

5. *Denial of paraphilic interest.* Confrontation of the patient's reported sexual interest versus his recorded visual reaction time interest follows a paradigm similar to that of confrontation using penile plethysmography results. When an individual denies, for example, having sexual interest in children but visual reaction time indicates high sexual interest, the individual is confronted with this discrepancy and, in many cases, admits his or her deviant sexual interests.

6. *Variation, duration, and quantity of visual reaction time measurement.* There is currently no standard methodology for measuring visual reaction time. Some systems have used the frequency of an operant response to maintain the opportunity to view a slide, comparing the time of attention to the stimulus category while carrying out a concomitant cognitive task with the time of attention to the slide category without the cognitive task. It is premature to determine which methodology will prove most effective in dealing with the sex offender population.[17,19]

7. *The relationship between visual reaction time in the office and the patient's behavior outside the office.* The problems in generalizing from sexual interest in the office to sexual behavior in the real world are as problematic for visual reaction time measurement as they are for penile plethysmography. Neither method can be used to verify that the individual assessed has actually acted on the sexual interest he or she displays in the office.

Polygraphy. Polygraphy is another physiological assessment method employed during initial assessment, treatment, posttreatment reassessment, and follow-up therapy. According to The Safer Society,[22] approximately 25% of treatment providers use polygraphy to assist in identifying the types and numbers of paraphilic acts the person has carried out before treatment or, more importantly, as a periodic means of verifying treatment compliance and/or posttreatment relapse (see Table 3–3). Polygraphs, like plethysmographs, do not meet the Frye standard for admissibility in court. However, they are a valuable adjunct to the clinical interview for gathering information regarding the person's behavior outside the treatment setting.[23]

Treatment for Persons With Paraphilia

The last 10 years has seen treatment for paraphilia focus on two primary areas: cognitive-behavior treatment and pharmacological treatment. In a recent survey by The Safer Society,[22] sex offender treatment providers were asked to identify the treatment components they employed. The results of this survey are listed in Table 3–3. Cognitive-behavior treatment has generally focused on

1. Behavior therapy to block or reduce inappropriate sexual arousal to deviant stimuli and to maximize or maintain nondeviant sexual arousal
2. Skills training to establish or expand prosocial skills
3. Changing cognitive distortions that the person has used to justify paraphilic behavior
4. The establishment of victim empathy; that is, a greater appreciation of the consequences of victimization
5. Relapse prevention—a methodology of organizing the various components of treatment so that the perpetrator, his family, the criminal justice system, and the therapist are all united in implementing treatment that minimizes the possibility of relapse

Behavior Therapy

Behavior therapies are implemented to help persons with paraphilias to block or reduce thoughts of, fantasies about, and urges toward deviant objects or behaviors so as to gain better control over their paraphilic behavior. Behavior therapies can be applied on an individual basis, but in the majority of large treatment programs in the United States treatments are applied in a group setting to improve the cost-effectiveness of the therapy. In nearly all cases, the behavior therapy is self-administered—that is, controlled by the patient. The patient is trained in the behavior therapy technique and then implements that therapy at home and makes an audiotape of the therapy product. These taped behavior therapy sessions are then reviewed in the group setting, with the therapist and other group members critiquing and advising the patient on how to make the treatment tapes more effective. The process then continues as the patients refine their behavior therapy skills and generate more tape recordings of behavior therapy sessions. Although it is not exhaustive, the list below represents behavior therapies commonly used in major programs.

Table 3–3. Treatment modalities used with adult sex offenders

Treatment modality	% of providers
Victim empathy	94.5
Anger/aggression management	92.0
Cognitive distortions	91.0
Relapse cycle	88.0
Social skills	88.0
Communication	88.0
Sex education	84.5
Personal victimization/trauma	84.5
Relapse prevention plan	83.5
Pre-assault/assault cycle	83.0
Relaxation techniques/stress management	82.5
Assertiveness training	81.5
Conflict resolution	79.0
Changing thinking errors (Samenow method)	78.0
Frustration tolerance/impulse control	77.5
Victim apology	75.0
Positive/prosocial sexuality	75.0
Journal keeping	73.5
Values clarification	69.0
Sexually transmitted disease	68.5
Alcoholics Anonymous	64.0
Sex role stereotyping	63.5
Autobiography	62.5
Employment/vocational issues	59.5
Dating skills	59.5
Relapse contract	53.5
Fantasy work	52.5
Narcotics Anonymous	52.5
Victim restitution	51.5
Reality therapy	51.0
Addictive cycle	49.0
Core relapse prevention group	46.0
Covert sensitization	38.5

(continued)

Table 3–3.   Treatment modalities used with adult sex offenders
          (continued)

Treatment modality	% of providers
Rational emotive therapy	37.5
Adult Child of Alcoholics	36.5
Sexaholics Anonymous	34.0
Polygraph	24.5
Masturbatory satiation	22.5
Masturbatory training	22.5
Sexual attitude reassignment	22.5
Modified aversive behavioral rehearsal	22.0
Verbal satiation	19.0
Experiential therapies	18.5
Art therapy	18.5
Masturbatory reconditioning	18.0
Dissociative state therapy	17.5
Sexual arousal measures/phallometry	17.0
Olfactory aversive techniques	16.5
Hypnosis	16.0
Minimal arousal conditioning	13.5
Sexual arousal card sorts	10.0
Biofeedback	7.5
Shaming	5.5
Faradic aversive techniques	3.0
Bodywork/massage therapy	2.5
Psychopharmacological agents	
Fluoxetine hydrochloride	31.5
Lithium carbonate	21.5
Minor tranquilizers	20.5
Major tranquilizers	19.0
Medroxyprogesterone acetate	19.0
Clomipramine hydrochloride	18.5
Buspirone hydrochloride	18.5
Serotonin reuptake inhibitors	12.0

Covert sensitization. Covert sensitization teaches the patient how to imagine the negative social consequences resulting from initial urges to become involved in paraphilic behavior.[24,25] Behavior does not occur in a vacuum. Nearly all behavior is preceded by thoughts, urges, and sometimes fantasies regarding possible behaviors that each of us could produce. As time passes, we elaborate on those urges and—sometimes—set in motion behaviors that increase the likelihood of implementation of an act. Persons with paraphilia find themselves under stress, affected by stimuli that they have seen, or in environments that in the past have led to deviant behavior. They sometimes then elaborate on prior experiences, begin to fantasize, and move toward situations in which the risk of perpetrating a paraphilic act increases markedly. Finally, they put themselves in proximity to a potential victim and, in many cases, carry out paraphilic acts.

Negative consequences of such paraphilic acts are infrequent, and paraphilic persons usually try not to think about the negative consequences of their behavior. During covert sensitization training, the patient imagines the chain of events that might lead to a paraphilic act, then imagines the most aversive social consequences to them, should they be discovered committing such an act. Numerous repetitions of the therapy teach the patient to become more and more adept at identifying his own antecedents to deviant behavior and pairing them with imaginable aversive consequences. Once the patient is adept at implementing the treatment technique, he implements the use of aversive scenes in the real world to block the chain of events leading to paraphilic acts.

Olfactory aversion. Some paraphilic persons are very adept at imagining covert scenes of aversive consequences and respond well to covert sensitization. Other paraphilic persons find it difficult to imagine such aversive scenes and are more responsive to olfactory aversion. This methodology is similar to covert sensitization, except that instead of using imaginable aversive scenes the patient learns to pair and associate the aversive consequence of smelling offensive odors to disrupt and block the chain of events leading to paraphilic acts. Ammonia (in the form of smelling salts) is the most commonly used offensive odor in such training, but other aversive odors have also been used. Ammonia aversion, like most of the behavior therapies, is patient-initiated and patient-implemented. Ammonia aversion has the added advantage that it is rather easy to implement any place, any time the patient's urges are high and need disruption. Maletzky[26] combined both covert sensitization and olfactory aversion to magnify the impact of each of the aversive therapy components.

Imaginable desensitization. Persons with a paraphilia frequently describe the sudden onset of powerful urges to act on their paraphilic behaviors. They see no other way of controlling these urges and the emotional stress they engender other than to engage in the paraphilic behavior. McConaghy[27] describes alternative methods for the paraphilic person to control these urges. The patient, with the assistance of the therapist, generates scenes that are capable of re-creating the situation of having strong paraphilic urges and the emotions and feelings associated with them. The patient is taught muscle relaxation methods and then imagines paraphilic scenes that are able to generate the types of urges that typically have led to his committing a paraphilic act. Once the emotions, feelings, and urges are sensed, the patient practices the relaxation methods to reduce his stress, rather than acting on those urges and feelings. Therapy is arranged so that increasingly more difficult situations and fantasies are imagined.

Modified aversive behavior rehearsal. A forerunner of modified aversive behavior rehearsal is described by Serber[28] and others. This is a treatment for paraphilic behaviors that can be enacted in the office setting without victimizing others (such as cross-dressing). The original therapy was described as shame aversion, intimating that its effective component was the shame produced in the person carrying out his paraphilic behavior in front of others, who gave him feedback on the ridiculousness of his behavior. More recently, there has been a shift away from the shame aversion components of this treatment and a greater focus on the cognitions or beliefs that the perpetrator has during the commission of paraphilic acts. Further modification has included videotaping the use of mannequins serving as victims of the perpetrator's deviant behavior. Smith and Wolfe,[29] for example, have pedophiles "molest" child mannequins, carrying out their typical pedophilic behavior while these acts are videotaped. Others have expanded these sessions to include the patient verbalizing his internal thoughts preceding these acts, and his beliefs regarding what the victim might be imagining or experiencing during the commission of the paraphilic act. These videotapes are then reviewed by the therapist, the patient, and other significant people, who evaluate how they see and/or experience the patient's victimization behavior. The net effect is not only the negative effects of being scrutinized closely by those viewing the simulated acts, but more importantly, an objective evaluation of the rationalizations and justifications used by paraphilic persons to excuse their behavior.

Satiation. The behavior and analytical literature hypothesizes that deviant arousal is maintained because the paraphilic person's deviant fantasies are repeatedly paired with the pleasure and enjoyment of orgasm, during both masturbation and the commission of paraphilic acts.[24] Marshall and Lippins[30] first described a method of treatment involving the patient masturbating to deviant fantasies for long periods of time to the point of boredom. This was later modified to instructing the patient to masturbate while fantasizing nondeviant fantasies to the point of ejaculation, and then to switch postorgasm to the use of deviant fantasy during masturbation, at a time when orgasm could not occur. Therefore, the use of deviant fantasy was associated with masturbation, but not with the pleasure of orgasm. In this way the use of deviant fantasies becomes disconnected from the pleasure and enjoyment of the masturbatory-orgasmic experience. Subsequent modifications have also incorporated the tape recording of such masturbatory sessions, so that they can be periodically checked to ensure compliance and accurate application of the treatment methodology.[24] In this controlled fashion, repeated use of the deviant fantasy satiates the patient so that the formerly highly erotic fantasy loses its erotic quality. It is also believed that the externalization of one's secret fantasies tends to destroy some of their erotic property.

Developing nonparaphilic arousal. Some—but certainly not all—persons with paraphilia fail to have adequate arousal to nonparaphilic themes. Approximately 7% of persons with pedophilia and a larger percentage of sadists, for example, fail to have sexual arousal devoid of paraphilic interests. Treatment to increase nonparaphilic arousal has been particularly problematic for therapists because strategies designed to develop nonparaphilic interest have been either unproductive or costly. Two procedures appear to hold the greatest promise for developing nonparaphilic interest. The first involves exposure—namely, having patients look at videotaped material depicting nondeviant stimuli, so that they can improve their skills at fantasizing nonparaphilic stimuli.[31]

A number of studies specifically recommend masturbatory conditioning, in which patients either masturbate exclusively to nonparaphilic themes[32,33] or gradually shift from deviant fantasy themes to incorporating progressively larger amounts of nondeviant fantasy.[34–37] Once the patients are able to use assisted nonparaphilic fantasy by looking at pictures of nondeviant themes, they shift the nondeviant stimuli to include individuals in their real world whom they find somewhat attractive, or at least not repulsive.

Training Prosocial Behaviors

Persons with a paraphilia may have had treatment to reduce paraphilic interests and/or to develop or increase nonparaphilic sexual interests, but they may still lack a variety of prosocial skills necessary to initiate or sustain a relationship with an adult partner. There is insufficient evidence to support the proposition that paraphilic behavior results from a lack of prosocial skills,[38] but in clinical practice a subset of paraphilic persons were found lacking in various prosocial behaviors.

Social skills training. Some persons with a paraphilia do not have the rudimentary skills necessary to initiate or maintain social interaction with an adult partner. They have not learned how to maintain eye contact, ask questions to move a social conversation along, or be nonthreatening in topics of conversation.[24] Social skills training involves the patient describing situations from his or her natural environment that have been problematic, analyzing how the conversation could be improved, and then, most importantly, role-playing behaviors that initiate or sustain conversation. The therapist provides positive feedback for the patient's successes. The patient then practices these skills in social situations outside of the office, returning with new situations that are problematic, to start the process over again.

Assertiveness training.   Assertiveness training is frequently provided to paraphilic persons who poorly modulate their assertiveness with others, frequently exploding with angry outbursts and harsh confrontations. Rapists, exhibitionists, and those who physically assault their adult partners frequently need assertive skills training. Other persons with a paraphilia need assertiveness training to overcome their passive style of interacting with others.

With this treatment patients learn to distinguish between aggressive, assertive, passive, and passive/aggressive responses and learn how to appropriately make requests for behavioral change in others. They also learn how to express their feelings and opinions and to ask for assistance from those in their environment. Role-playing is the pivotal component of assertiveness training, providing patients with numerous opportunities to practice situations that have occurred in their environment when they were unable to assert themselves or unsuccessful at doing so.

Anger management training.   Anger management training is provided to paraphilic persons who have difficulty appropriately coping with their anger. Some persons with a paraphilia tend to overcontrol their anger, whereas others are in denial that they ever even experience anger. Others are unable to modulate their anger and frequently explode in angry outbursts. Anger management training focuses on helping the patient identify the antecedents or triggers to his anger, recognize his typical response to anger and realize how he learned this response, learn appropriate ways to express his anger, and, most importantly, identify ways that he can reduce his risk of experiencing excessive anger in the future.[39] There is frequent role-playing of appropriate coping techniques with the therapist or other group members, who provide feedback to the patient.

Sex education and/or sexual dysfunction training. Some persons with a paraphilia lack basic sexual knowledge or have specific sexual dysfunctions that impede their potential for appropriate sexual interaction with adult partners. Fetishists, transvestites, and some pedophiles become so involved in their paraphilic behavior that either they fail to develop appropriate sexual knowledge and skills, or else their preoccupation with their paraphilic behavior leads to their losing the skills they once had. Training involves not only basic sex education but also the specifics of sexual communication and learning to develop the closeness and intimacy with a potential sexual partner that could lead to a sexual interaction.

Cognitive training. Persons with paraphilia, like all of us, attempt to rationalize and justify their inappropriate behavior. When an exhibitionist, for example, sees the surprised, startled embarrassment or laughter on the face of the person to whom he has exposed himself, that person's response may conflict with his fantasy about the person's reaction. Since the exhibitionist leaves immediately after exposing himself and does not talk to his victim, he tends to rationalize and incorporate the victim's response (irrespective of what it is) to fit his own cognitive beliefs about the person's mental state in response to his behavior. For example, he may reinterpret the victim's surprise as her being impressed by the size of his penis. The victim's smile or laughter might be misinterpreted as signs of the pleasure she received from seeing his penis. The victim looking over her shoulder as she exits the situation to get away from him may be misinterpreted by the exhibitionist as further evidence of her wanting to see his penis or his erection. Or he may have some other interpretation that satisfies his own interpretation of this being a positive experience for the victim. Rapists, for example, may interpret the victim's failure to report the rape as evidence that the rape was an enjoyable experience for her. Rapists frequently believe that women find it difficult to assert themselves sexually. Rapists believe that victims say no to sexual advances not because they do not want to have sex but because they want to avoid the guilt they would feel for complying with sexual activity. Pedophiles justify their actions by stating that they were only providing sex education to the child or by contending that their act was not child molestation because it only involved fondling the child; or they minimize the importance of their behavior by noting that they did not use physical force. Pedophiles frequently rationalize that they are staunch believers that all individuals, including children, can decide whether they wish to be sexual, and that unless the child specifically says he or she does not want to be sexual, the child is consenting to the pedophilic behavior.[40–42]

Surprisingly, the cognitive distortions and rationalizations of one paraphilic person may be startlingly different from those of another, even within the same category of paraphilia. This is because the cognitive distortions of paraphilic persons are highly idiosyncratic and develop on an individual basis, without feedback from others. Therapy involves externalizing the patient's justifications and rationalizations for his or her inappropriate sexual behavior and mobilizing other persons with a paraphilia to confront these distortions and point out their illogical nature.

Victim empathy training. An important aspect of treatment involves modifying the patient's beliefs about the consequences of his or her behavior to the victim. Since most paraphilic persons exit the scene of their paraphilic behavior or are not present when the emotional consequences of their behavior have their impact on the victim, most persons with a paraphilia fail to appreciate the negative consequences that their behavior has on their victims. Victim empathy training[43] involves the patient reviewing videotapes in which victims of paraphilic behavior describe the impact of the victimization and its personal consequences to them. People with paraphilia are also provided with written descriptions of paraphilic acts from the victim's perspective. The paraphilic persons are then asked to write descriptions of their acts from their vantage point and then, later, from the vantage point of the victim. Feedback from other paraphilic group members and the therapist help them appreciate how victims experience such victimization and how the consequences to the victim are in sharp contrast to the perpetrator's view of the victimization experience.

Maintaining therapeutic gains/relapse prevention. Most behavior therapies involve the patients learning treatment modalities that they can implement any time in the future when urges to relapse are strong. Virtually no treatment assumes that once it is provided the patient is cured, never to have subsequent paraphilic urges. It is important, therefore, to have maintenance strategies to anticipate the individual's subsequent urges and a treatment plan to block or stop those urges anywhere, anytime. Maintenance of the patient's therapeutic progress is inhibited when there is a lack of communication between the therapist and the patient's family, those in the patient's environment, and the patient's parole or probation officer. The blocking of such communication emanates in part from the stance that the psychiatrist takes; that is, not to talk with others regarding problems discussed with the patient. In other words, the tradition of not communicating directly with those other than the patient appears to reduce continuity of care and protection of possible future victims, thereby increasing the likelihood of relapse and incarceration of the patient.

A further block to communication with those in the patient's family and environment sometimes results from the family and others not wanting to know what the person has done, thereby maintaining their denial of the patient's problem. A third block emanates from territorial issues, when psychiatrists and probation or parole officers do not communicate with each other as a result of their attempts to maintain their respective territories. A further block emanates from the paraphilic person not wanting others to be informed of his paraphilic behavior and interests.

Unfortunately, these various communication blocks appear to harm everyone involved in such cases. Patients suffer because of their increased risk of recidivism, loss of self-esteem, incarceration, and disruption of their family and personal lives. Potential victims lose when they are victimized. The family of the patient suffers when they learn of the patient's relapse and sometimes subsequent incarceration. Such consequences are exceedingly disruptive to the lives of patients' families. Parole or probation officers lose when someone they are responsible for supervising relapses. Since they have been given the legal responsibility for supervising such a case, relapses are seen, in part, as a failure to supervise adequately. Psychiatrists suffer a sense of failure because they too had hoped for treatment to effectively stop the perpetrator's relapsing.

Surveillance groups. Given the severe consequences to all of relapse, treatment must include specific organized communication between all parties involved. This will reduce the risk of reoffense by opening up communication so that everyone can participate in the process of supervision. Abel and Rouleau[25] describe the development of surveillance groups and a surveillance system. Five individuals from the patient's environment—at least one each from his family, work, and social contacts—participate in a meeting with the therapist in which the patient explains in detail the extent of his paraphilic behavior and situations that in the past increased the risk of his carrying out paraphilic acts. In so doing, the patient takes responsibility for his paraphilic acts but also trains those in his environment to identify behaviors that in the past were antecedent to relapse. A surveillance form evolves from this meeting. All members of the surveillance group complete a checklist of these high-risk situations and forward it to the therapist twice a month, thereby increasing the number of participants in the supervisory network in order to identify early behaviors to which the therapist and others should be more attentive.

Relapse prevention. Relapse prevention is an extensive framework for carrying out the supervisory process. Based on strategies originally developed to prevent relapse in substance abusers,[44] this model has now been extended to relapse prevention specifically designed for sex offenders.[45] Relapse prevention is based on the assumption that sex offenders make the decision during treatment that they will abstain from committing paraphilic behaviors. As a result, persons with paraphilia have high expectations of successfully coping with urges to commit sex crimes. Having made the assumption that abstinence will prevent subsequent behavior, the paraphilic person then makes what appears to be an inconsequential decision. This apparently irrelevant decision, nonetheless, leads him into a high-risk situation. These high-risk situations frequently involve stress related to interpersonal conflicts or negative emotional states. The paraphilic person, being unprepared to cope with that stress or emotional conflict, engages in thoughts and behaviors that lead to a lapse, such as placing himself in a situation where he has offended in the past or looking at individuals who provoke his paraphilic interests. Sensing that the lapse is contrary to his decision for abstinence, the perpetrator loses self-esteem, sees himself as failing, and devalues himself—a response referred to as the abstinence violation effect. The reduction in self-esteem and sense of failure increase the risk for further lapses and, eventually, a relapse of the deviant behavior.[46-48] The relapse prevention model[48] involves 1) the patient developing a number of strategies to prevent this sequence of events, including strategies to prevent lapses from turning into relapses by the use of cognitive restructuring; 2) a maintenance plan anticipating high-risk situations and implementing strategies to effectively avoid and/or cope with these situations; 3) contracting that sets a limit on what lapses are allowed to occur before the therapist is notified immediately; 4) maintenance manuals; and 5) relapse rehearsal.

Summary

Paraphilic interests are surprisingly common in the general population. Those who most frequently seek psychiatric care for sex offenses are those accused of or involved in child molestation, voyeurism, exhibitionism, fetishism, frottage, and public masturbation. Although some sex offenders commit crimes exclusively in one category of paraphilic behavior, a surprisingly high number of paraphilic persons have previously been involved or are currently involved in different paraphilias with victims of both genders and of various ages. The psychiatrist's evaluation of arrest records, the clinical psychiatric interview, and paper-and-pencil testing assist in understanding some paraphilic persons, but many times the patient's denial necessitates additional evaluation with psychophysiological methods that evaluate the patient's sexual interest, using penile plethysmography, visual reaction time assessment, and/or polygraphs.

Treatment of paraphilic behavior has been extensively investigated in the last 10 years and generally includes cognitive-behavior treatment with a strong focus on relapse prevention and the use of medications to reduce sexual drive, including medroxyprogesterone acetate and, more recently, serotonin reuptake inhibitors. Maintenance therapy is especially important to ensure a coordinated effort to help paraphilic persons control their inappropriate behavior. The combined efforts of the patient, the patient's family, the probation or parole officer, the patient's friends, and the therapist are all vital components of this coordinated effort. The increasing utilization of sexual drive–reducing agents has brought the psychiatrist into a vital position of assisting in the patient's successful treatment.

References

1. Crepault C, Coulture M: Men's erotic fantasies. Arch Sex Behav 9:565–580, 1980
2. Templeman TL, Stinnett RD: Patterns of sexual arousal and history in a "normal" sample of young men. Arch Sex Behav 10:137–150, 1991
3. Abel GG, Becker JV, Mittelman MS, et al: Self-reported sex crimes of non-incarcerated paraphiliacs. Journal of Interpersonal Violence 2:3–25, 1987
4. Abel GG, Osborn CA: Stopping sexual violence. Psychiatric Annals 22:301–306, 1992
4a. Abel GG, Osborn CA: The paraphilias: the extent and nature of sexually deviant and criminal behavior, in Psychiatric Clinics of North America. Edited by Bradford JMW. Philadelphia, PA, WB Saunders, 1992, pp 675–687
5. Salter AC: Treating Child Sex Offenders and Victims: A Practical

Guide. Newbury Park, CA, Sage, 1988, pp 182–205

6. Kercher G, Long L: Supervision and Treatment of Sex Offenders. Huntsville, TX, Sam Houston Press, 1991, pp 53–72

7. Zuckerman M: Physiological measures of sexual arousal in the human. Psychol Bull 25:297–327, 1971

8. Freund K: Phallometric diagnosis with "non-admitters." Behav Res Ther 17:451–457, 1979

9. Murphy WD, Barbaree HE: Assessments of Sexual Offenders by Measures of Erectile Response: Psychometric Properties and Decision Making. Washington, DC, National Institute of Mental Health, 1988

10. Laws DR, Rubin HB: Instructional control of an autonomic response. J Appl Behav Anal 2:93–99, 1969

11. Abel GG, Lawry SS, Karlstrom EM, et al: Screening tests for pedophilia. Criminal Justice and Behavior 21:115–131, 1994

12. Abel GG: Behavioral treatment of child molesters, in Perspectives on Behavioral Medicine. Edited by Stunkard AJ, Baum A. New York, Erlbaum, 1989, pp 223–242

13. Freund K: Assessment of pedophilia, in Adult Sexual Interest in Children. Edited by Cook M, Howells SK. New York, Academic Press, 1981, pp 139–179

14. Rosenzweig S: The photoscope as an objective device for evaluating sexual interest. Psychosom Med 4:150–157, 1942

15. Amoroso D, Brown M, Pruesse M, et al: The effects of physiological measurement and presence of others on ratings of erotic stimuli. Canadian Journal of Behavioural Science 4:191–203, 1972

16. Brown M, Amoroso D, Ware E, et al: Factors affecting viewing time of pornography. J Soc Psychol 90:125–135, 1973

17. Love R, Sloan L, Schmidt M: Viewing pornography and sex guilt: the priggish, the prudent and the profligate. J Consult Clin Psychol 44:624–629, 1976

18. Ware E, Brown M, Amoroso D, et al: The semantic meaning of pornographic stimuli for college males. Canadian Journal of Behavioural Science 4:204–209, 1972

19. Wright L, Adams H: Assessment of sexual preference using a choice reaction time task. Journal of Psychopathology and Behavioral Assessment 16:221–231, 1994

20. Zamansky H: A technique for measuring homosexual tendencies. J Pers 24:436–448, 1956

21. Abel G, Huffman J, Warberg B, et al: Visual reaction time and plethysmography as measures of sexual interest in child molesters. Sexual Abuse: A Journal of Research and Treatment (in press)
22. Freeman-Longo RE, Bird S, Stevenson WF, et al: Nationwide Survey of Treatment Programs and Models. Brandon, VT, Safer Press, 1994, pp 19–20
23. Abrams S, Abrams JB: Polygraph Testing of the Pedophile. Portland, OR, Ryan Gwinner Press, 1993
24. Abel GG, Becker JV, Cunningham-Rathner J, et al: The Treatment of Child Molesters. Atlanta, GA, Behavioral Medicine Institute of Atlanta, 1984
25. Abel GG, Rouleau JL: Male sex offenders, in Handbook of Outpatient Treatment of Adults. Edited by Thase ME, Edelstein BA, Hersen M. New York, Plenum, 1990, pp 271–290
26. Maletzky BM: Self-referred versus court-referred sexually deviant patients: success with assisted covert sensitization. Behavior Therapy 11:306–314, 1980
27. McConaghy N: Assessment and treatment of sex offenders: the Prince of Wales Programme. Aust N Z J Psychiatry 24:175–181, 1990
28. Serber M: Shame aversion therapy. J Behav Ther Exp Psychiatry 1:213–215, 1970
29. Smith TA, Wolfe RW: A treatment model for sexual aggression. Journal of Social Work and Human Sexuality 7:149–164, 1988
30. Marshall WL, Lippins K: The clinical value of boredom: a procedure for reducing inappropriate sexual interests. J Nerv Ment Dis 165:283–287, 1977
31. Barlow DH, Agras WS, Abel GG, et al: Case histories and shorter communications. biofeedback and reinforcement to increase heterosexual arousal in homosexuals. Behav Res Ther 13:45–50, 1975
32. Kremsdorf RB, Holman ML, Laws DR: Orgasmic reconditioning without deviant imagery: a case report with a pedophile. Behav Res Ther 18:203–207, 1980
33. Maletzky BM: Orgasmic reconditioning, in Dictionary of Behavior Therapy Techniques. Edited by Bellack AS, Hersen M. New York, Pergamon, 1985, pp 157–158
34. Abel GG, Blanchard EB, Barlow DH, et al: A case report of the behavioral treatment of a sadistic rapist. Paper presented at the Ninth Annual Convention of the Association for the Advancement of Behavior Therapy, San Francisco, CA, December 1975

35. Conrad SH, Wincze JP: Orgasmic reconditioning: a controlled study of the effects upon the sexual arousal and behavior of adult male homosexuals. Behavior Therapy 7:155–166, 1976

36. Marques J: Orgasmic reconditioning: changing sexual object choice through controlling masturbation fantasies. J Behav Ther Exp Psychiatry 1:263–271, 1970

37. Leonard SR, Hayes SC: Sexual fantasy alternation. J Behav Ther Exp Psychiatry 3:241–249, 1983

38. Okami P, Goldberg A: Personality correlates of pedophilia: are they reliable indicators? Journal of Sex Research 29:297–328, 1992

39. Cullen M, Freeman-Longo RE: Men and Anger: A Relapse Prevention Guide to Understanding and Managing Your Anger. Brandon, VT: The Safer Society Press, 1995

40. Abel GG, Mittelman M, Becker JV: Sex offenders: results of assessment and recommendations for treatment, in Clinical Criminology: The Assessment and Treatment of Criminal Behavior. Edited by Ben-Aron MH, Hucker SJ, Webster CD. Toronto, M and M Graphics, 1985, pp 191–205

41. Lange A: Rational-Emotive Therapy: A Treatment Manual. Tampa, FL, Florida Mental Health Institute, 1986

42. Murphy WD: Assessment and modification of cognitive distortions in sex offenders, in Handbook of Sexual Assault: Issues, Theories and Treatment of the Offender. Edited by Marshall WL, Laws DR, Barbaree HE. New York, Plenum, 1990, pp 331–342

43. Knopp FH: Retraining Adult Sex Offenders: Methods and Models. Syracuse, NY, The Safer Society Press, 1984

44. Marlatt GA: Feeding the PIG: the problem of immediate gratification, in Relapse Prevention With Sex Offenders Laws. Edited by Laws DR. New York, Guilford, 1989, pp 46–62

45. Pithers WD, Marques J, Gibat CC, et al: Relapse prevention with sexual aggressives: a self-control model of treatment and maintenance of change, in The Sexual Aggressor: Current Perspectives on Treatment. Edited by Greer JG, Stuart IR. New York, Van Nostrand Reinhold, 1983, pp 214–239

46. Pithers WD: Relapse prevention with sexual aggressors, in Handbook of Sexual Assault: Issues, Theories and Treatment of the Offender. Edited by Marshall WL, Laws DR, Barbaree HE. New York, Plenum, 1990, pp 343–361

47. Pithers WD, Kashima KM, Cumming GF, et al: Relapse prevention:

a method of enhancing maintenance of change in sex offenders, in Treating Child Sex Offenders. Edited by Salter AC. Newbury Park, CA, Sage, 1988, pp 131–170

48. Pithers WD, Kashima KM, Cumming GF, et al: Relapse prevention of sexual aggression. Ann N Y Acad Sci 528:244–260, 1998

Further Readings

Marshall WL, Barbaree HE: Oucome of comprehensive cognitive-behavioral treatment programs, in Handbook of Sexual Assault: Issues, Theories and Treatment of the Offender. New York, Plenum, 1990, pp 363–385

Furby L, Weinrott MR, Blackshaw L: Sex offender recidivism: a review. Psychol Bull 105:3–30, 1989

Pithers WD: Treatment of rapists: reinterpretation of early outcome data and exploratory constructs to enhance therapeutic efficacy, in Sexual Aggression: Issues in Etiology, Assessment, and Treatment. Edited by Nagayama-Hall R, Hirschman R, Graham JR, et al. Washington, DC: Taylor & Francis, 1993, pp 167–196

CHAPTER 4

Juvenile Sex Offenders

Although there is a considerable body of clinical and research literature on adult sex offenders, there has been a relative paucity of data on juvenile sex offenders until the past decade. The reasons for the lack of focus on juvenile sex offenders range from the belief that all sexual behavior by juveniles is exploratory to concern about giving a juvenile a label of paraphilia. Although as mental health professionals we need to be cautious about mislabeling normal sexual behavior as abnormal and further stigmatizing adolescents by applying psychiatric labels, conversely we do need to address, assess, and treat youths who engage in sexual behavior that is age inappropriate and that involves coercion or lack of consent.

The legal definition of sexual abuse is fairly straightforward but narrow in scope. Sexual abuse of a child is generally defined by statute as involving sexual assault against a minor, and the law often specifies a minimum age difference between the victim and perpetrator, such as 5 years. Sexual assault is usually defined as knowingly inflicting sexual penetration, intrusion, or contact on a victim involving conditions of physical force, threats, or other means of coercion.

Kempe[1] defines sexual abuse as the involvement of dependent, developmentally immature children and adolescents in sexual activities that they do not fully comprehend, to which they are unable to give informed consent, or that violate the social taboos of family roles. Researchers have generally required that sexual experiences be unwanted, forced, or coercive in order to be categorized as sexually abusive.[2]

Sexual abuse of children by adults is usually easy to define based on the nature of the behaviors and the age differences, although assessment is frequently difficult because of factual disputes. Age and behavior are often inadequate factors by themselves in determining the presence or absence of sexual abuse when the sexual interactions involve youths under age 18. There is generally no difficulty in determining that sexual abuse has occurred when an older adolescent engages in sexual activity with a small child, but health care professionals have had difficulty in distinguishing between "normal" sexual experimentation and sexually abusive behavior among similarly aged children or adolescents, especially when the behavior is characterized by minimal intrusiveness and/or aggressiveness. A more thorough evaluation under the latter circumstances is required concerning issues related to consent and the dynamics of the relationship between the youths.[3,4]

Informed consent in this context generally requires that a person be adequately informed and competent to make a decision about participating in the sexual activity and that the decision be a voluntary one. Various ages have arbitrarily been legally assigned as indicating presumed competence to make a decision about involvement in sexual relationships. The issue of voluntariness is often difficult to assess because of the wide range of coercive techniques used by perpetrators in sexual abuse situations. Sexual activity occurring through mutual agreement and negotiation is very different from sexual behavior that is the result of deception, enticement, entrapment, intimidation, or physical force. Sexually abusive behavior is often characterized by a significant lack of equality in the relationship between the juveniles. Factors to be considered in assessing the equality include the physical, cognitive, and emotional development of each child.[4]

The nature of the sexual activity and the circumstances of the sexual contact are significant factors to evaluate in the assessment of sexual abuse. Sexual acts that appear to reflect more advanced knowledge or experience than would be expected for the age of the involved persons may be a sign of sexual abuse. Sexual activity perceived as a way of hurting, embarrassing, degrading, punishing, or controlling someone should raise suspicion concerning probable abuse.[5] Sexual interactions in which one individual disregards the needs and desires of the other individual are usually experienced as abusive. Bolton and colleagues[6] proposed an abuse of sexuality model that emphasizes psychosocial and sociocultural experiences that may also be perceived as sexual victimization without overt sexual contact.

Available statistics indicate that a substantial number of sex offenses are committed by juveniles. Estimates suggest that 20% of all rapes and between 30% and 50% of child molestations are perpetrated by male adolescents.[7]

Studies of adult offenders reveal that a significant proportion of persons with a paraphilic disorder developed their deviant sexual arousal patterns before age 18.[8-10] Groth[11] refuted earlier findings, which tended to minimize the deviant sexual behavior of male adolescents, characterizing it as reflecting either experimentation or innocent sexual activities. Findings by Becker et al.[7,12] that the mean onset of nondeviant genital sexual behavior preceded the onset of deviant sexual behavior in 22 male adolescents support the assessment that deviant sexual behavior is not the exploration of the inexperienced.

The number of sexual offenses committed by an offender dramatically increases as adulthood is reached. A study of 240 adult offenders, who had all experienced their deviant sexual arousal before age 18, reported that each offender averaged 581 attempted or completed deviant sexual acts. Their average of 380 victims per offender was more than 56 times the number of victims per offender for adolescent sex offenders.[8] Longo and Groth[9] reported that at least one of three convicted adult rapists or child molester showed progression from nonviolent sex crimes during adolescence to more serious sexual assaults as adults.

Several extensive reviews of the characteristics of juvenile offenders can be found in the psychological and psychiatric literature.[13-15] Available data indicate that juvenile sex offenders are a heterogeneous population. Ryan et al.[16] summarized information obtained from the National Adolescent Perpetrator Network Uniform Data Collection System (UDCS), which contains data for over 1,600 juveniles referred for evaluation and/or treatment to 90 sex offender–specific programs in 30 states. This database indicates that juvenile sex offenders range in age from 5 to 19 with a median age between 14 and 15. These juveniles represent all racial, ethnic, and socioeconomic classes. Forty-two percent of the subjects had a history of physical abuse, 39% were known to have been sexually abused, and neglect was documented in 26%. Twenty-five percent of the sexually abused subjects reported that their perpetrator was less than 5 years older than themselves. Sixty percent of the juveniles had penetrated their victims, and in 90% of cases, the juvenile perpetrators knew the victims.

The UDCS revealed that the average number of victims known at the time of evaluation was 7.7, with 39% being blood relatives of the young offender from the same household. Sexual abuse of a peer accounted for 10% of the offenses; sexual victimization of strangers constituted only 6%; and only 4.5% of the sexual abuse victims were adults. These findings are consistent with those reported by Becker et al.[12] and Fehrenbach and Monastersky[17] Almost 70% of the referring offenses involved anal or vaginal penetration and/or oral-genital contact. Ninety percent of the juvenile offenders were male and 10% were female. In 90% of cases, the victims were known to the juvenile perpetrators.[16]

There are no generally accepted models or theories that explain the etiology of youthful sex offending, although theorists from several schools of psychopathology have attempted to explain the etiology of deviant sexual behavior and interests.[14]

A model proposed by McCloskey and Figueredo[18] has recently received partial support.[19] This model proposes a graded continuum of sexual tactics used by men, ranging from the coerciveness of subtle social pressure to overtly violent assault. Violence is seen as instrumental in the pursuit of sexual gratification as opposed to a behavioral end in itself. Kobayashi et al.[19] tested a theoretical model utilizing data on 117 juvenile male sex offenders who had been referred from either criminal justice or social service agencies to a clinic that treated juvenile sex offenders. The theoretical model that was tested included several family factors, including perceived parental deviance, history of child sexual and physical abuse, and children's bonding to their parents. Adolescent sex offenders who had been physically abused by their fathers and sexually abused by a male perpetrator were found to have increased sexual aggression. Children's bonding to their mothers was found to decrease their sexual aggression. These findings speak to the issue that male typical sexual and aggressive behavior will be modeled on that of available male models (e.g., father or other significant males) and that "normal bonding" to the mother (or other significant women) served affiliative and prosocial needs, thereby decreasing sexual aggression. Further research is warranted on this proposed theoretical model. Although this model's focus is on male adolescents, it remains to be seen whether it is applicable to female adolescents and prepubescent offenders.

Efforts to establish topologies for youthful sex offenders are ongoing. Two taxonomic systems have been proposed,[20,21] but neither has been experimentally validated.

Although a considerable amount of knowledge has been gained on youthful sex offenders during the past decade, many questions remain to be answered.

Medicolegal Issues

There is general agreement that protection of the community through the prevention of sexual abuse is a very high priority of intervention and that community safety takes priority over any other conflicting consideration when treating adolescent sex offenders.[22] The clinician should be familiar with and responsive to the relevant requirements for reporting to child protective services or the equivalent state agency. The adolescent and his parents should be informed about these requirements and criminal justice issues related to the limits of confidentiality before beginning the assessment process. It is often advisable for the adolescent to have legal counsel in order to decide about making new disclosures of additional offenses during assessment and/or treatment so the implications of such disclosures are clearly understood by the adolescent and/or his legal guardian. Guardians ad litem are often appointed by the court in certain jurisdictions to represent the best interest of the adolescent in such matters.

Prosecution should be a component of *most* interventions in juvenile sex offenses for a variety of reasons, including community safety, deterrence, and increased probability that the adolescent will participate in treatment through the use of the legal system. Prosecution reinforces the fact that a victim has suffered harm and may offer incentive for the offender to change. Appropriate legal intervention helps pierce the denial often present in the adolescent by demonstrating to him that he will be held accountable for his behavior. The juvenile court, which has significantly changed its focus and process since its creation in 1899, has a range of options available that include dismissal, diversion, probation, and a variety of placement options, including residential treatment, training school, and psychiatric hospitalization.[23,24]

Court-ordered probation and/or parole conditions that require participation in an offense-specific treatment program are generally necessary to prevent adolescent offenders from prematurely leaving treatment. Some families of adolescent sex offenders may need dependency and neglect petitions filed in order to mandate participation and/or cooperation with treatment. Probation officers and court workers should have specific training for working with this population and the treatment team. They should act promptly (e.g., file violations on offenders) when an adolescent is not following mandated conditions.[22]

Diversion programs, deferred prosecution, and deferred sentencing are other legal responses that can serve a therapeutic purpose if treatment is mandated and closely supervised with clear legal consequences for the offender if he does not follow specified conditions. Plea bargaining to a nonsexual charge is strongly discouraged, because it often supports the offender's denial and may prevent participation in the necessary offense-specific intervention.[22]

Treatment should be coordinated with appropriate law enforcement personnel, the judicial system, child protective services, educators, parents, and other persons involved with the adolescent offender. This interagency approach to sexual abuse treatment can be facilitated before the adolescent is admitted into a treatment program by having the adolescent and his legal custodian sign a waiver of confidentiality that allows the clinician(s) to provide information to other appropriate professionals who are involved with the adolescent.

Assessment

The assessment of adolescent sex offenders is often a complicated and time-consuming process related to clinical, logistic, and legal issues. There are at present no scientifically validated instruments to classify sex offenders, although useful guidelines concerning evaluation and treatment issues have been published.[5,22,25,26] The National Task Force on Juvenile Sexual Offending[22] has developed guidelines for the following six types of evaluations:

1. Pretrial (investigative)
2. Presentencing (dangerousness/risk; placement/prognosis)
3. Postadjudication clinical assessment; treatment issues/modes
4. Needs (treatment planning and progress in treatment)
5. Release /termination from treatment program (community safety and successful application of treatment tools)
6. Monitoring and follow-up

The investigative evaluation is generally carried out by law enforcement and child protective agencies. Referrals for evaluation during the pretrial phase may be precipitated by clinical and/or legal issues. The adolescent and his family may need crisis intervention related to their initial involvement with social services and/or the police. The adolescent's attorney may request an evaluation in order to receive assistance for a variety of legal purposes, such as recommendations concerning diversion programs, placement, and treatment.

Pretrial assessments are often a good opportunity—especially when the factual circumstances surrounding the sexual offense are very clear—to obtain accurate and relevant history from the alleged offender and his family. They are likely to be more open during such assessments if they perceive that the process may help the adolescent avoid incarceration. However, it is not unusual for the adolescent and/or his family to deny or minimize participation in inappropriate sexual behavior for many reasons, including an attempt to avoid legal consequences. Under such circumstances, the evaluation will not be very helpful during this phase because of the unreliability of the history.[27] Issues related to the limits of confidentiality, reporting requirements, and the purpose(s) of the evaluation should be clearly explained to both the adolescent and his family before beginning the assessment process.

Presentencing evaluations are often requested to provide the court with a comprehensive assessment of the adolescent that addresses issues including diagnosis, prognosis, potential dangerousness, and placement and treatment recommendations. More factual information is generally available from the criminal justice system regarding the events surrounding the sexual offense(s) at the time of these evaluations. A guilty verdict will often reduce the adolescent's denial, which will result in his providing more useful information.

Risk assessment, which is a component of the presentencing evaluation, addresses the potential dangerousness of the youth because of sexually abusive and/or other behaviors. There are currently no validated scientific instruments or criteria to assess the risk of reoffense. Clinical experience and a comprehensive evaluation provide the basis for such risk assessments, which have a strong impact on placement decisions. Placement recommendations should be consistent with the least restrictive environment that allows for community safety. When the victim and perpetrator live in the same home, out-of-home placement for the perpetrator is generally required to provide an environment for the victim that is both emotionally and physically safe.

A comprehensive adolescent sex offender assessment should include the following factors:[4,5,22,27,28]

- Victim's statements (as obtained from police and social services reports, mental health professionals, and the like)
- Background information (including family, educational, medical, psychosocial, and developmental histories)
- Interpersonal relationship history
- Sexual history (including categories of deviant sexual interest and progression of sexually aggressive behavior over time)
- Reported use of sexually deviant fantasies and interests
- Intensity of sexual arousal during time surrounding each offense
- Dynamics/process of victim selection
- Use of coercion, force, violence, and weapons
- Behavioral warning signs
- Identifiable triggers leading to inappropriate sexual behaviors
- Thinking errors (e.g., cognitive distortions, irrational thinking)
- Spectrum of injury to the victim (e.g., violation of trust, creation of fear, physical injury)
- Sadistic elements
- Ritualistic/obsessive characteristics
- Deviant nonsexual interest
- History of assaultive behavior
- Issues related to separation/loss
- Antisocial characteristics
- Psychiatric diagnosis (e.g., disruptive behavior disorders, affective disorders, developmental disorders, personality disorders, posttraumatic stress disorder, substance abuse disorder, organic mental disorder)
- Ability to accept responsibility
- Degree of denial or minimization
- Understanding wrongfulness
- Concern for injury to victim
- Quality of social, assertive, and empathic skills
- Family's response (e.g., denial, minimization, support, ability to intervene appropriately)

- Exposure to pornography
- History of victimization (sexual, physical, or emotional)
- Ability to control deviant sexual interest
- Knowledge and expression of appropriate sexual desire
- School performance/educational level
- Mental status examination

These assessments require multiple interviews with the adolescent offender and should include interviews with his parents. It is helpful to interview the parents both separately and together to obtain a developmental history of the adolescent and a relevant background history of each parent. The parents' response to the adolescent's offense, their ability to supervise and availability for supervision, family attitudes regarding sexual issues, family system dynamics, and the parents' attitude about the need for treatment are essential factors to assess. A history of sexual abuse within the adolescent's family, problems in decision making, problems in expression of emotions, family secrets, role reversals, boundary problems, and various intrafamilial alliances are commonly present.[22,25,27,29] Discrepancies between the adolescent's self-reporting and information obtained from parents and/or other sources need to be explored and further understood.

The evaluator should also be knowledgeable about and sensitive to cultural issues. Culture is an important factor to consider in understanding sexually aggressive youths and their families and communities, although culture sensitivity does not equate to acceptance of abusive behavior.[22]

Community safety requirements and the adolescent's clinical state and/or legal status will usually determine the setting for these assessments. An inpatient psychiatric evaluation may facilitate completion of a comprehensive evaluation in a relatively brief period of time, although such a setting is not very cost-effective. These time-consuming and complicated assessments are generally best performed over longer time frames for many reasons, including the time required to establish a working relationship with the adolescent and his family and difficulties obtaining information from other agencies. Interviewing the adolescent during several different time frames can provide the evaluator with information relevant to coping skills and credibility issues. A residential treatment setting may offer many of the advantages of an inpatient psychiatric unit without the associated costs.

Psychological tests can be helpful in assessing the needs of specific offenders, although it is generally agreed that an adolescent's sexual offending behavior does not constitute a single homogeneous class of behavior.[30] Some psychometric tests that have been used include a number of sexual self-reporting measures, such as the Adolescent Sexual Interest Cardsort[31] to determine the presence of deviant sexual interests; the Adolescent Cognition Scale[32] to assess the presence of any distorted cognitions regarding sexual behaviors (however, it should be noted that the cognition scale did not discriminate between an adolescent sex offender and non–sex offender groups); and the Matson Evaluation of Social Skills in Youngsters,[33] which is designed to assess the social and assertive skills of adolescents. Other tests that measure personality characteristics (e.g., Minnesota Multiphasic Personality Inventory,[33a] Thematic Apperception Test[33b]) and intellectual functioning (e.g., Wechsler Intelligence Scale for Children, Revised) can provide useful information concerning an individual offender.

Plethysmography (phallometric assessment of physiological sexual arousal by use of equipment that measures penile circumference in males) is a potentially useful technique in the evaluation of some sexually abusive youths, although this issue is controversial.[22,34–36] The controversy includes issues related to informed consent, concerns about exposing adolescents to deviant sexual stimuli, and the reliability, validity, and predictive power of phallometric testing.[22,37,38] Phallometric testing can be helpful in providing a baseline of the individual's sexual arousal and assessing the efficacy of treatment employed to alter sexual arousal or interest patterns.[39,40] It is recommended that practitioners using phallometric assessment adhere to the standardized procedures for use of the equipment developed by the Association for the Treatment of Sexual Abusers[41] and be consistent with guidelines developed by the National Task Force on Juvenile Sexual Offending.[22]

The postadjudication clinical assessment, which should be performed before entry into any level of treatment, may require only an assessment update if a presentencing evaluation has been completed and has been made available to the treatment provider. The principles summarized above for the presentencing evaluation should be followed. The presentencing evaluation and/or the postadjudication clinical assessment will provide a structure for the initial treatment plan. Ongoing evaluation during the treatment process is required to reformulate the treatment plan as more information about the adolescent is obtained. The range of deviant sexual behavior and levels of violent ideation are usually not fully disclosed until much later in the treatment process.[3]

Assessment for purposes of determining changes in placement and/or termination from treatment programs should be based on specific measurable objectives, observable changes, and demonstrated ability to apply changes in current situations. Areas to be assessed include[22]

- Acknowledgment of the responsibility for offenses (e.g., use of denial, minimization, or projection of blame)
- Ability to identify contributing factors to offending cycle
- Resolution of contributing factors to sexually abusive behavior
- Demonstration of empathic thinking
- Capacity to manage stress and adequately handle negative feelings
- Positive interpersonal relationships
- Ability to identify and maintain control of deviant sexual arousal
- Resolution of personal victimization and/or loss issues
- Ability to communicate and understand behavior patterns in the treatment environment and to utilize this information outside the therapy setting
- The family's ability to recognize risk factors and to help the adolescent manage differently and seek help

Monitoring and follow-up assessments are designed to evaluate the adolescent's current situation and reinforce the tools acquired by him during treatment in order to minimize the risk of relapse. Assessments, using a relapse prevention model, will monitor the offender for signs of[22,42]

- Return to high-risk behavior
- Irresponsible decision making
- Use of denial or minimization
- Substance use
- Use of pornography or deviant fantasy
- Placement failure
- Decompensation/regression

Treatment

All communities should strive to offer a continuum of care for youthful sex offenders, from outpatient treatment to day treatment to residential treatment. Whereas in 1982 there were only 22 identified treatment programs in the United States for juvenile offenders, there are at present more than 800—the majority being community based.

Following a comprehensive assessment an individualized treatment plan should be developed for the youthful offender. Treatment should be specific and structured and may include individual therapy, group therapy, family therapy, and adjunctive therapies (e.g., substance abuse and psychopharmacological treatment).

Treatment modalities that have been commonly used include individual and group cognitive-behavior therapies, psychoeducational interventions, family therapies, biological therapies, and relapse prevention models.

The National Task Force on Juvenile Sexual Offending[22] recommends that treatment address the following areas:

- Denial, minimization, and projecting of blame
- Accountability for all abusive or exploitive behaviors
- Thinking errors/irrational thinking
- Factors contributing to cycle of abuse behavior
- Apparently irrelevant or unrelated decisions that set up a high-risk situation
- History of offending behavior
- Self-responsibility in sexual and nonsexual functioning
- Irresponsible decision making/high-risk behaviors
- Empathy development/victim personalization
- Long-term management of sexually deviant impulses
- Power and control behaviors/covert exploitation
- History of client's own victimization
- Life history/autobiography
- Helplessness and lack of control
- Delusions of persecution
- Impulsivity and poor judgment
- Anger management and frustration tolerance
- Feeling identification and management
- Values clarification, including victim empathy
- Ability to experience pleasure in nonexploitive activities
- Substance abuse/addictive behaviors
- Self-esteem and identity
- Arousal patterns/deviant fantasizing
- Positive sexual development/identity
- Sex education/sexually transmitted disease including AIDS
- Sex-role stereotyping
- Cultural influences
- Sexual identity issues; homosexuality/homophobia
- Communication/social skills training
- Assertiveness training
- Dating/relationship building

- Employment/vocational issues
- Family dysfunction and sibling issues
- Educational issues

It is critical that the juvenile's family members be assessed and provided treatment to determine if there are any factors within the home that may have been causative or that continue to reinforce the behavior. Thomas[29] proposed a five-stage model that outlines the work to be done as part of the family component of adolescent sex offender treatment. Stage I includes working with the crisis of disclosure, stage II is to conduct a thorough assessment of the family that includes demographics, family environment, historical data, abuse history, psychological data, family background, developmental and medical histories of the offender, medical and developmental histories of the family, educational histories, sexual histories, leisure time, legal history of family members, and substance abuse history. Thomas notes that it is also important to determine the family members' perceptions of the sexual abuse, the reaction of the family to disclosure, and the reactions of extended family members. Stage III involves family therapy interventions, setting goals, and planning. Issues to be addressed include denial, minimization and projection of blame, lack of empathy, abusive power and powerlessness, anger management, blurring of role boundaries, human sexuality, divided loyalty, and substance abuse. Stage IV involves reconstruction and reunification of the family; stage V is termination and aftercare.

Becker and Kaplan[35] describe a multicomponent treatment based on a cognitive-behavior model. The majority of treatment is conducted in a group format and includes the following components: verbal satiation, covert sensitization, cognitive restructuring, social skills training, anger management, and sex education. Values clarification treatment is carried out over a 10-month period. These authors report a 9% sexual recidivism rate at 12 months' follow-up.

Gray and Pithers[42] discuss the use of a relapse prevention model with sexually aggressive youths. Relapse prevention focuses on facilitating internal self-management skills. Youths are taught awareness of the seemingly unimportant decisions (SUDs) that they make; high risk factors; abstinence; violation effects; and coping strategies. A relapse prevention model relies heavily on an external, supervisory dimension. Basically a "prevention team" is established that works collaboratively with the juvenile to help him diminish the potential for reoffending.

Borduin et al.[43] have conducted the only recent controlled therapy outcome study with adolescent sex offenders. These authors randomly assigned juvenile sex offenders to one of two conditions, multisystemic therapy or individual therapy. Follow-up ranged from 21 to 49 months, with an average period of 37 months. The recidivism rate for those who received multisystem therapy was 12.5% compared with a recidivism rate of 75% for those who received individual therapy.

Although there has been a dearth of published follow-up studies on youthful sex offenders, several researchers have identified factors associated with recidivism. Schram et al.[44] identified four factors associated with sexual recidivism in treated adolescent offender populations: 1) having deviant sexual arousal patterns, 2) a history of truancy, 3) thinking errors, and 4) having had at least one prior conviction for a sexual offense.

Smith and Monastersky[45] identified five factors associated with recidivism: 1) lack of understanding of the exploitive nature of their offense, 2) inability to identify their personal strengths, 3) unhealthy attitudes toward sexuality (not understanding their own sexuality), 4) failure to understand the seriousness of the sexual offense, and 5) unwillingness to discuss and explore the offense in a nondefensive manner.

Summary and Recommendations

There has been a relative paucity of data on juvenile sex offenders until the past decade due to both myths about adolescent sexual perpetrators and concerns regarding stigmatization. Available statistics suggest that male adolescents perpetrate 20% of all rapes and between 30% and 50% of child molestations. The juvenile perpetrator generally has multiple victims, with most offenses involving anal or vaginal penetration and/or oral-genital contact.

Available data indicate that juvenile sex offenders are a heterogeneous population. One large study indicates that juvenile sex offenders range in age from 5 to 19, with a median age between 14 and 15. It is very common for a juvenile sex offender to have been the victim of physical or sexual abuse and/or neglect.

It is important that these youths receive treatment to help them deal with both their own victimization and perpetration problems. In the course of assessment and treatment it is essential to consider community safety issues. The clinician should be familiar with and responsive to the relevant requirements for reporting to child protective services or the equivalent state agency.

Legal involvement should be a component of most interventions in adolescent sex offenses for a variety of reasons, including community safety, deterrence, and increased probability that the adolescent will participate in treatment through the use of the legal system. The use of probation, parole, deferred prosecution, or diversion can be a useful legal response for such purposes.

The limit of confidentiality should be clearly explained to the adolescent and his parents or legal guardian before initiating a psychiatric evaluation and/or treatment. The assessment of adolescent sex offenders is often a complicated and time-consuming process related to clinical, logistic, and legal issues. These assessments require multiple interviews with the adolescent offender and should include, when possible, interviews with his parents.

All communities should strive to offer a continuum of care for youthful sex offenders, from outpatient treatment to day treatment to residential treatment. Treatment should be specific and structured and may include individual therapy, group therapy, family therapy, and adjunctive therapies (e.g., substance abuse and psychopharmacological treatment).

Treatment modalities that have been commonly used include individual and cognitive-behavior therapies, psychoeducational interventions, family therapies, biological therapies, and relapse prevention models.

Future clinical research needs to focus on 1) identification of the developmental pathways to sexual offending, 2) empirically derived typologies, and 3) controlled treatment outcome studies with long-term follow-ups. Finally, efforts must be made to develop primary and secondary prevention strategies.

References

1. Kempe CH: Incest and other forms of sexual abuse, in The Battered Child, 3rd Edition. Edited by Kempe CH, Helfer RE. Chicago, IL, University of Chicago Press, 1980, pp 198–214
2. Peters D, Wyatt GE, Finkelhor D: Prevalence, in Sourcebook on Child Sexual Abuse. Edited by Finkelhor D. Newbury Park, CA, Sage, 1986, pp 15–59
3. Ryan GD: Juvenile sex offenders: defining the population, in Juvenile Sexual Offending: Causes, Consequences, and Corrections. Edited by Ryan GD, Lane SL. San Francisco, CA, Jossey-Bass, 1997, pp 3–9
4. Metzner JL, Ryan GD: Sexual abuse perpetration, in Conduct Disorders in Children and Adolescents. Edited by Sholevar GP. Washington, DC, American Psychiatric Press, 1994, pp 119–144
5. Groth AN, Loredo CM: Juvenile sexual offenders: guidelines for assessment. International Journal of Offender Therapy and Comparative Criminology 25:31–39, 1981
6. Bolton FG, Morris LA, MacEachron AE: Males at Risk: The Other Side of Sexual Abuse. Newbury Park, CA, Sage, 1989
7. Becker JV, Kaplan M, Cunningham-Rathner J, et al: Characteristics of adolescent incest perpetrators: preliminary findings. Journal of Family Violence 1:85–97, 1986
8. Abel G, Rouleau J, Cunningham-Rathner J: Sexually aggressive behavior, in Psychiatry and Psychology: Perspectives and Standards for Interdisciplinary Practice. Edited by Curran W, McGarry A, Shah S. Philadelphia, PA, FA Davis, 1986, pp 289–314
9. Longo RE, Groth AN: Juvenile sexual offenses and the histories of adult rapists and child molesters. International Journal of Offender Therapy and Comparative Criminology 27:150–155, 1983
10. Marshall WL, Barbaree HE, Eccles A: Early onset in deviant sexuality in child molesters. Journal of Interpersonal Violence 6:323–336, 1991

11. Groth AN: The adolescent sex offender and his prey. International Journal of Offender Therapy and Comparative Criminology 21:249–254, 1977

12. Becker JV, Cunningham-Rathner J, Kaplan MS: Adolescent sexual offenders: demographics, criminal and sexual histories, and recommendations for reducing future offenses. Journal of Interpersonal Violence 1:431–445, 1986

13. Becker JV, Harris CD, Sales RD: Juveniles who commit sex offenses: a critical review of research, in Sexual Aggression: Issues in Etiology and Assessment, Treatment, and Policy. Edited by Hall GCN, Hirschman R, Graham J, et al. Washington, DC, Taylor and Francis, 1993

14. Pithers WD, Becker JV, Kafka M, et al: Children with sexual behavior problems, adolescent sex abusers, and adult sex offenders: assessment and treatment, in American Psychiatric Press Review of Psychiatry. Edited by Oldham JM, Riba MB. Washington, DC, American Psychiatric Press, 1995, pp 779–818

15. Morenz BM, Becker JV: The treatment of youthful sexual offenders. Applied and Preventive Psychology 4:247–256, 1995

16. Ryan G, Miyoshi TJ, Metzner JL, et al: Trends in a national sample of sexually abusive youths. J Am Acad Child Adolesc Psychiatry 35:17–25, 1996

17. Fehrenbach PA, Monastersky C: Characteristics of female adolescent sexual offenders. Am J Orthopsychiatry 58:148–151, 1986

18. McCloskey LA, Figueredo AJ: Sex, money and paternity: evolutionary psychology of domestic violence. Journal of Ethology and Sociobiology 14:353–379, 1993

19. Kobayashi J, Sales BD, Becker JV, et al: Perceived parental deviance, parental-child bonding, child abuse and child sexual aggression. Sexual Abuse: A Journal of Research and Treatment 7:25–44, 1995

20. O'Brien M, Bera W: Adolescent sexual offenders: a descriptive typology. A Newsletter of the National Family Life Education Network 1:1–5, 1986

21. Knight RA, Prentky RA: Exploring characteristics for classifying juvenile sex offenders, in The Juvenile Sex Offender. Edited by Barbaree HE, Marshall WL, Hudson SM. New York, Guilford, 1993, pp 45–83

22. National Task Force on Juvenile Sexual Offending: The revised report from the National Task Force on Juvenile Sexual Offending,

1993 of the National Adolescent Perpetrator Network. Juvenile and Family Court Journal 44:1–120, 1993

23. Schetky DH, Benedek EP: History of child forensic psychiatry, in Clinical Handbook of Child Psychiatry and the Law. Edited by Schetky DH, Benedek EP. Baltimore, MD, Williams & Wilkins, 1992, pp 1–3

24. Kalogerakis MG: Juvenile delinquency, in Clinical Handbook of Child Psychiatry and the Law. Edited by Schetky DH, Benedek EP. Baltimore, MD, Williams & Wilkins, 1992, pp 191–215

25. Otey EM, Ryan GD (eds): Adolescent Sex Offenders: Issues in Research and Treatment (DHHS Publ No ADM-85–1396). Rockville, MD, U.S. Department of Health and Human Services, 1985

26. Wenet G, Clark T: Juvenile Sexual Offender Decision Criteria. Seattle, WA, Juvenile Sexual Offender Program, University of Washington Adolescent Clinic, 1984

27. Ryan G, Metzner JL, Krugman RD: When the abuser is a child, in Understanding and Managing Child Sexual Abuse. Edited by Oates KR. Sydney, NSW, Australia: Harcourt Brace Jovanovich, 1990, pp 258–274

28. Stevenson HC, Wimberley R: Assessment of treatment impact of sexually aggressive youth. Journal of Offender Counseling, Services and Rehabilitation 15:55–68, 1990

29. Thomas J: The adolescent sex offender's family in treatment, in Juvenile Sexual Offending: Causes, Consequences and Corrections. Edited by Ryan GD, Lane SL. San Francisco, CA, Jossey-Bass, 1997, pp 360–403

30. Smith WR, Monastersky C, Deisher RM: MMPI-based personality types among juvenile sex offenders. J Clin Psychol 43:422–430, 1987

31. Hunter JA, Becker JV, Goodwin DW, et al: The Adolescent Sexual Interest Cardsort: test-retest reliability and concurrent validity. Arch Sex Behav 24(5):555–561, 1995

32. Hunter JA, Becker JV, Kaplan MS, et al: The reliability and discriminative utility of the Adolescent Cognition Scale for juvenile sex offenders. Annals of Sex Research 4:281–286, 1991

33. Matson JL, Esveldt-Dawson K, Kazdin A: Evaluating social skills with youngsters. J Clin Child Psychol 12:174–180, 1983

33a. Hathaway SR, McKinley JC: Minnesota Multiphasic Personality Inventory, Revised. Minneapolis, MN, University of Minnesota, 1970

33b. Murray HA: Thematic Apperception Test. Cambridge, MA, Harvard University Press, 1971

33c. Wechsler D: Wechsler Intelligence Scale for Children, Revised. New York, Harcourt Brace Jovanovich, 1974

34. Travin S, Cullen K, Melella JT: Use and abuse of erection measurements: a forensic perspective. Bulletin of the American Academy of Psychiatry and the Law 16:235–250, 1988

35. Becker JV, Kaplan MS: Cognitive behavioral treatment of the juvenile sex offender, in The Juvenile Sex Offender. Edited by Barbaree HE, Marshall WL, Hudson SM. New York, Guilford, 1993, pp 264–277

36. Hunter JA, Becker JV: The role of deviant sexual arousal in juvenile sexual offending: etiology, evaluation and treatment. Criminal Justice and Behavior 21(1):132–149, 1994

37. Saunders EB, Awad GA: Assessment, management and treatment planning for male adolescent sexual offenders. Am J Orthopsychiatry 58:571–579, 1988

38. Murphy WD, Krisak J, Stalgaitis S, et al: Use of penile tumescence measures with incarcerated rapists: further validity issues. Arch Sex Behav 13:545–554, 1984

39. Becker JV, Kaplan MS: The assessment of sexual offenders. Advances in Behavioral Assessment of Children and Families 4:97–118, 1988

40. Hunter JA, Goodwin DW: The clinical utility of satiation therapy with juvenile sexual offenders: variations and efficacy. Annals of Sex Research 5:71–80, 1992

41. Association for the Treatment of Sexual Abusers: Ethical Standards and Principles for the Management of Sexual Abusers. Beaverton, OR: Association for the Treatment of Sexual Abusers, 1997, pp 44–51

42. Gray AS, Pithers WD: Relapse prevention with sexually aggressive adolescents, in The Juvenile Sex Offender. Edited by Barbaree HE, Marshall WL, Hudson SM. New York, Guilford, 1993, pp 289–320

43. Borduin CM, Henggeler SW, Blaske DM, et al: Multisystemic treatment of adolescent sexual offenders. International Journal of Offender Therapy and Comparative Criminology 34:105–113, 1990

44. Schram DD, Malloy CD, Rowe WE: Juvenile sex offenders: a follow-up study of reoffense behavior. Interchange (Newsletter on the National Adolescent Perpetrator Network) July 1992, pp 1–3

45. Smith WR, Monastersky C: Assessing juvenile sex offenders and preventing the cycle of abuse. Journal of Child Care 3:115–140, 1986

CHAPTER 5

Pharmacological Treatment of Sex Offenders

The pharmacological treatment of sex offenders is based on certain assumptions. One approach is based on the theory that suppression of the sexual drive will result in a decrease in paraphilic behavior. It assumes that a reduction in sexual drive will also reduce the fantasies and urges that accompany a paraphilia (e.g., pedophilia). The aim of this treatment approach would be to produce an asexual individual in whom both nondeviant and deviant sexual behavior are suppressed. A more ideal outcome would be to eliminate the paraphilic behavior while leaving nonparaphilic sexual behavior intact. Thus, a second and preferable aim of pharmacological treatment would be to suppress the deviant sexual fantasies, urges, and behavior but to allow the sex offender to remain sexually active in a nondeviant manner.

Other theories that affect the pharmacological treatment of the paraphilias are those that include them either in the obsessive-compulsive spectrum of disorders or in impulse control disorder.[1-3] In these cases, the deviant sexual behavior as well as the paraphilic fantasies and urges are experienced as ego-dystonic. If this theoretical framework is adopted, then paraphilic urges are analogous to compulsions and paraphilic fantasies to obsessions. This theoretical approach is supported by the response of a variety of paraphilias to pharmacological agents used in the treatment of obsessive-compulsive disorder (OCD). These same drugs appear to be effective in the treatment of some impulse control disorders such as kleptomania.[4] The aim of this pharmacological approach fits the second aim of treatment, the suppression of deviant elements of fantasy, urges, and behavior while allowing nondeviant sexual behavior to exist.

Biological treatments, specifically surgical castration and stereotaxic neurosurgery,[5] have been used in sex offenders to reduce their sexual drive and to prevent recidivism. Stereotaxic neurosurgery, because of the level of intrusiveness, has been used infrequently and is only of theoretical interest. Sex offenders treated by surgical castration, which is intrusive and irreversible, constitute a heterogeneous group. Usually the procedure is performed on only the most serious offenders—those who victimize women and children (i.e., rapists and those with pedophilia). These offenders also appear to have serious personality disorders and other difficulties such as alcoholism, although good studies of the actual comorbidity of psychiatric disorders in this group are lacking. Surgical castration is important because it mediates sexual behavior by suppressing the sexual drive. It accomplishes this by reducing testosterone levels, as do the antiandrogens. In addition, postcastration follow-up studies[6–11] provide the most comprehensive outcome data on the effect of reducing plasma testosterone and the resultant suppression of the sexual drive and attendant deviant sexual behavior (Table 5–1). These studies[6–13] have reported recidivism rates of less than 5% with follow-up periods up to 20 years in large numbers of sex offenders. These studies involved mainly perpetrators of the most serious of the paraphilias: rape (sexual sadism) and pedophilia.[9,11,12] These outcome studies of surgical castration provide the theoretical basis for pursuing a pharmacological treatment approach to the paraphilias that is based on a reduction of testosterone.

Testosterone is the principal androgen produced by the testes in most animal species. It strongly influences both male and female sexual drive and the resultant sexual behavior.[14] In animal studies, the higher the level of evolution of the species, the less direct the in-

Table 5–1. Recidivism rates following castration

Study	Follow-up period (years)	N	Pre rate (%)	Post rate (%)
Langeluddeke 1963[6a]	20	1,036	84	2.3
Cornu 1973[6b]	5	127	76.8	4.1
Bremer 1959	5–10	216	58	2.9
Sturup 1968, 1972[10,11, note a]	30	900		2.2

Note. Pre rate, recidivism rate before castration; post rate, recidivism rate after castration.
[a]Mostly rapists.
Source. Data from Heim and Hursch 1979;[7] Bradford and Pawlak 1987.[48]

fluence of hormones on sexual behavior, although sexual behavior remains androgen dependent regardless of the species.[15] Animal studies show that male copulatory behavior is almost entirely dependent on circulating levels of plasma testosterone.[16] These effects are mediated through action on intracellular androgen receptors in target organs.[17] The various target organ cells respond according to their genetic complement.[17] Testosterone is metabolized to dihydrotestosterone (DHT), which binds to the androgen receptors.[18] Androgen synthesizing cells have receptors for luteinizing hormone (LH), which is the tropic hormone for testosterone production.[19] Testosterone is also converted to estrogens in the brain and may then act through the estrogen receptors.[20] In the male, testosterone is also responsible for fetal androgenization.[21] It is the binding of the hormone to the receptor that results in the biological response. This binding to the receptor sites can be inhibited by competitive and noncompetitive mechanisms. Competitive inhibitors act by combining with the receptor so that the steroid molecule cannot be bound. Noncompetitive inhibition decreases the number of receptor sites. The sensitivity of the androgen receptors in the central nervous system (provided there is sufficient testosterone above a specific individually determined threshold) determines male sexual behavior patterns.

The androgen receptors are found in the various androgen-sensitive target organs—such as the prostate[17] and various parts of the brain, including the limbic system and the anterior hypothalamus—where they respond to testosterone.[17] The antiandrogen and the hormonal treatment approaches target a reduction of available androgen at the receptor level. The effect of surgical castration is to globally reduce available androgen by the removal of the testes, where approximately 95% of the available testosterone in the body is produced. The mechanism of action of the antiandrogens (e.g., cyproterone acetate) and the hormonal agents (e.g., medroxyprogesterone acetate [MPA] and estradiol) is more complex. However, there is a reduction of available androgen, principally testosterone, as well as secondary effects on sexual behavior.[16] The behavioral effects of testosterone are the result of its action on the brain, although the actual principal site of action is a matter of some debate.[14] In humans aggression, including sexual aggression, appears to be testosterone dependent.[22–32]

The pharmacological treatment of sex offenders is therefore based mostly on sexual drive suppression by a variety of pharmacological agents. The most common pharmacological treatments are antiandrogens, hormonal agents without a specific antiandrogen profile, and other pharmacological agents.

Antiandrogens

Cyproterone Acetate

Cyproterone acetate (CPA) has antiandrogenic, antigonadotropic, and progestational effects.[33] Its principal mode of action is on the androgen receptors, where it blocks the intracellular uptake of testosterone and the intracellular metabolism of the androgen.[33–35] The effects are largely dose dependent, and the effects on sexual behavior are correlated with a reduction of plasma testosterone. Erections, ejaculate, and spermatogenesis are all decreased. Sexual fantasies are suppressed or completely eliminated. Animal studies have shown that CPA can affect the onset of puberty as well as fetal development and differentiation.[36]

CPA has a strong progestational action.[34] It also has a specific antigonadotropic effect similar to that of other progestogens.[34,36] The "pure antiandrogens," specifically cyproterone and the nonsteroidal agent flutamide, have no antigonadotropic effects. This means that in CPA, it is the acetate radical that gives a progestational action. CPA blocks or reduces the secretion of luteinizing hormone–releasing hormone (LH-RH).[36] The full antigonadotropic effect of CPA is exercised only in women, because in men the antiandrogenic and antigonadotropic effects balance out. The specific mode of action of CPA is competitive inhibition of testosterone and DHT at specific androgen receptor sites. CPA is 100% bioavailable orally with a plasma half-life of 38 ± 5 hours. The injectable form reaches maximum plasma level in 82 hours. Oral dosage varies from 50 to 200 mg daily, whereas parenteral dosage is 200–400 mg every 1–2 weeks.

There are some possible risks to CPA treatment, but these are highly unlikely to occur at the dosage levels used to treat the paraphilias. There is the possibility of liver dysfunction and adrenal suppression[35,37] as well as feminization, manifesting as temporary or protracted gynecomastia.

Many patients treated with CPA report a feeling of calm as a result of the treatment. This appears to be specifically related to a reduction of anxiety and irritability.[38] This reduction in irritability appears to be part of a general reduction in psychopathological symptoms found during treatment with CPA.[38]

Laschet and Laschet[39] reported the first clinical studies of CPA from Germany. More than 100 paraphilic men, primarily exhibitionists but also pedophiles and sexual sadists, 50% of whom were also sexual offenders, were treated for periods of least 6 months to more than 4 years. In about 80% of cases 100 mg CPA per day eliminated sexual drive, erections, and orgasm, whereas 50 mg/day reduced libido but allowed erections to occur. Parenteral CPA was administered at 300 mg biweekly. In about 20% of exhibitionists there was a complete elimination of all deviant behavior even after treatment with CPA was terminated. Some undesirable side effects were also seen. These were fatigue; transient depressive moods; weight gain (in about 20% of patients, presenting only after

6 months of treatment); reduced body hair; increased scalp hair; slight gynecomastia; decreased sebaceous gland secretion; and reduced spermatogenesis. Laschet and Laschet[40] reported on 300 men treated for up to 8 years with very good responses. Minimal side effects with long-term management were reported. Davies[41] reported on 50 patients treated with CPA for up to 5 years. This was a heterogeneous sample of hypersexual men, which included patients with schizophrenia, elderly patients, and mentally handicapped patients. All patients showed improvement in sexual behavior. Only minimal side effects were reported. Bancroft and co-workers[42] completed a study on 12 patients comparing CPA (100 mg/day) and ethinyl estradiol (0.2 mg/day) and found that both drugs reduced sexual interest, activity, and arousal. There were few significant side effects, although relatively more were noted with ethinyl estradiol. One patient taking CPA developed a severe depressive episode and had to be withdrawn from the study. CPA reduced plasma testosterone, follicle-stimulating hormone (FSH), and LH, whereas estradiol caused increased levels of testosterone and LH.

Other studies of CPA treatment[41,43–46] have also shown that CPA is effective in reducing deviant sexual behaviors in a variety of men with paraphilia. Most of these were open, uncontrolled trials.

The largest group of sexually deviant men ($N = 547$) treated with CPA, who would most likely fit DSM-III-R or DSM-IV definitions of paraphilic disorder, were reported on jointly by Mothes et al.[45] and Laschet and Laschet.[40] Laschet and Laschet[40] reported a detailed analysis of 100 of these patients and a study of a further 200. The duration of treatment was from 2 months to 8 years. The dosage ranged from 50 to 200 mg/day for oral administration, whereas depot CPA was given at either weekly or biweekly intervals in dosages ranging from 300 to 600 mg per injection. Unwanted side effects observed in the first 2 months included fatigue, hypersomnia, depression, negative nitrogen balance, and weight gain. By 3 months the nitrogen balance had returned to normal, as had calcium and phosphate metabolism. At approximately 8 months, in up to 20% of patients, there were some signs of feminization, as evidenced by gynecomastia and a reduction of body hair associated with an increase in scalp hair. Beneficial responses affecting paraphilic behavior were decreases in erections, sexual fantasies, and sexual drive in 80% of the patients treated with 100 mg/day of CPA orally. The response was reported as being due to the antiandrogen effect of CPA. Subsequently 25 patients were followed for up to 5 years after treatment without any recurrence of paraphilic behavior. In contrast, paraphilia associated with organic brain damage responded only partially to treatment with CPA, whereas nonsexual aggressive behavior did not appear to respond to it at all.

Three studies, a double-blind placebo crossover study,[38] a study of the effects of CPA on the sexual arousal patterns of persons with pedophilia,[47] and a single case study[48] with repeated measures all demonstrated that CPA was an effective agent in the treatment of the more severe paraphilias, specifically sexual sadism and pedophilia. The single case study[48] was interesting in that it involved the treatment of a patient with severe sadistic homosexual pedophilia and very severe temporal lobe brain damage. The response to CPA was assessed with a variety of measures, which included sexual arousal responses. For the first time a differential outcome on the pattern of sexual arousal was seen. This was also seen in the study on the sexual arousal patterns of pedophiles treated with CPA.[47] CPA reduced deviant sexual arousal (i.e., pedophilic arousal and sadistic arousal) while having less impact on the nondeviant arousal responses (e.g., arousal to consensual sex with adult women). Thus, a normalization of the sexual arousal responses was seen: deviant sexual arousal was suppressed while nondeviant arousal was left intact or was enhanced.

A double-blind placebo crossover study of CPA was conducted on 19 patients, including 12 men with pedophilia who were also sex offenders with high pretreatment recidivism rates (mean = 2.5 previous convictions per offender).[38] All the subjects met the DSM-III-R criteria for a paraphilia. Measure of self-reported sexual activity showed a significant reduction on CPA. CPA[38] significantly decreased other objective measures of sexual drive, such as sexual fantasies and masturbation frequency.

Cooper et al.[49] reported on a double-blind, placebo-controlled study of CPA and MPA with a two-dose comparison format. The duration of the study was 28 weeks. Both drugs appeared equally effective in reducing fantasies, morning erections, masturbation, and level of sexual frustration. Sexual arousal responses were all reduced, but in a variable way. The expected hormonal effects were seen.

Cooper and colleagues[50] reported on a single case of pedophilia receiving long-term treatment with CPA. The patient was studied in detail for over 3 years. The active drug (compared with times when the patient was being given a placebo and when no treatment was administered) reduced sexual arousal and sex hormones. Prolactin levels were increased. When CPA was discontinued, all measures returned to pretreatment levels in 3 weeks.

It is clear that CPA can play an important role in the treatment of sex offenders. It is well documented that, in some men with paraphilia and some sex offenders, it can substantially reduce recidivism rates and that these beneficial effects continue even when treatment is terminated (Table 5–2). This also means intermittent

Table 5–2. Recidivism rates following treatment with cyproterone acetate (CPA)

Study	Follow-up period (years)	N	Pre rate (%)	Post rate (%)[a]
Horn 1973[50a]	1–4.5	33	100	0
Baron et al. 1977[50b]	1	6	50	0
Fahndrich 1974[50c]	3	14	93	0
Davies 1974[41]	3	16	100	0
Appelt and Floru 1974[55a]	1.5	6	100	16.7
Jost (1974)[55b]	4	10	100	0
Jost (1975)[55c]	3	11	54	0

Note. Pre rate, recidivism rate before CPA treatment; post rate, recidivism rate after CPA treatment.
[a]Corrections made for patient compliance, inadequate dosage, and inadequate information on relapse.
Source. Data from Ortmann 1980;[9] Bradford and Pawlak 1987.[48]

long-term pharmacological treatment, rather than continuous treatment, can be used with CPA.

Other Antiandrogens

Other antiandrogens, such as the nonsteroidal agent flutamide (which is used in the treatment of carcinoma of the prostate), may also be effective in the treatment of the paraphilias.

Hormonal Agents Without a Specific Antiandrogen Profile

Estrogens

Hormonal agents, starting initially with estrogens, have also been used for reduction of sexual drive and treatment of sexual offenders.[51-54] Side effects are a contraindication to their use today.

Phenothiazines

Several studies have reported that a number of different phenothiazines reduce sexual drive and sexually deviant behavior. Benperidol, a butyrophenone, has been described as having a specific effect.[55,56] A study by Tennent et al.[57] compared benperidol, chlorpromazine, and a placebo and found that benperidol was significantly more effective in reducing sexual interest than either of the other two agents. Most neuroleptics have some antilibidinal effect, although the exact mechanism of action is not fully understood. These agents should not be used in the primary treatment of a paraphilia; however, if sexually deviant behavior presents secondarily to a major psychiatric disorder, then a suitable neuroleptic would be the treatment of choice. In these cases it is likely that the paraphilic behavior became manifest as a result of disinhibition, rather than being instances of true paraphilia, unless the symptoms of deviance were present prior to the development of the psychosis. There is very little difference between the various agents in these circumstances, because whatever controls the psychosis should suppress the deviant sexual behavior.

Medroxyprogesterone Acetate

Medroxyprogesterone acetate (MPA) is the hormonal agent that has received the most attention in the treatment of sex offenders in North America. The first study[58] showing that MPA reduces the sexual drive in men was reported in 1958. Money[59] described the first instance of the use of MPA in treating sexual deviancy. Following this, a number of studies[49,60–70] were conducted using MPA for the treatment of sexually deviant men.

The principal mechanism of action of MPA is through the induction of testosterone-A-reductase in the liver. This enhances the metabolic clearance of testosterone and reduces plasma levels of testosterone.[71] In addition, MPA has an antigonadotropic effect. It is questionable if it has any effect in competing with the androgens at the androgen receptors and is therefore not a true antiandrogen.[71] It also affects the binding of testosterone to the plasma testosterone-binding globulin.

There are some potential side effects of MPA treatment that have to be considered. Walker and Meyer[69] reviewed published and unpublished data on MPA and reported on a number of these. Although they found no evidence of blood pressure changes or alterations in routine serum biochemistry, they did report weight gain (in approximately 50% of subjects); decrease in sperm production (this returned to normal levels after 6 months of treatment); a hyperinsulinemic response to a glucose load; and gallbladder and gastrointestinal dysfunction. There was also reported to be a reversal of any testicular atrophy that might have occurred. Some patients reported a worsening of headaches, and there was a single case of diabetes mellitus. Gagne[64] and Berlin and Meinecke[63] also reported similar side effects. However, desirable effects on sexual functioning were observed, including reductions in sexual drive, erotic fantasies, sexual activity, and possibly aggressiveness.[72] Money et al.[73] reported that the effect on aggressive behavior appeared to be a placebo-like response.

With few exceptions, the clinical studies of MPA that have been reported are open trials. Money[59,67,74] provided the first clinical reports of the use of MPA in the treatment of a variety of paraphilias.

Wiedeking et al.[70] reported on the treatment of 11 impulsive and sexually deviant XYY males for 1 year.

In a study of the treatment of exhibitionists, Langevin et al.[65] compared MPA to assertiveness training. Because there was a high dropout rate, this study's findings are of limited validity.

Berlin and Meinecke[63] treated 20 men with a variety of paraphilias with MPA. Three of the patients relapsed while taking MPA, and 10 of the 11 patients relapsed after discontinuing MPA against medical advice. MPA in this study appeared to be an effective treatment provided there was compliance with treatment. There was a high relapse rate with noncompliance.

Gagne[64] combined MPA with milieu therapy for a period of 12 months. He reported on the outcome with 48 patients, the largest group of whom was homosexual pedophiles. The treatment regimen was aimed at keeping plasma testosterone at less than 250 ng/100 mL. The patients received 200 mg intramuscularly three times per week in the first 2 weeks; 200 mg once or twice per week for the next 4 weeks; and then either 100 mg per week or 200 mg every 2 weeks as maintenance treatment. Forty patients improved substantially, and this was maintained throughout the follow-up period, although the length of follow-up is not given.

A single case study of the use of MPA to treat a patient with hypersexual pedophilia[75] during 18 months showed a positive treatment response.

Wincze and colleagues[76] used MPA in the treatment of three recidivist pedophiles in a single-case experimental design with a double-blind procedure in place for the administration of the medication. The three single-case studies were combined for the report. They included sexual arousal tests, including penile tumescence and nocturnal penile tumescence. They noted significant reduction in sexual arousal to erotic stimuli. Nocturnal penile tumescence was also significantly reduced.

Kiersch[62] studied the use of MPA in eight subjects. Four of the subjects completed a 64-week follow-up period. The effectiveness of treatment response was measured by self-report and sexual arousal measures, with each patient acting as his own control subject. MPA was given at 400 mg/week for 16 weeks, alternating with saline injections for a crossover period of 16 weeks. The results were extremely variable, and the study was flawed because of the extremely long half-life of MPA.

Meyer et al.[61] studied 40 men treated with MPA and with group and individual therapy. The paraphilias varied (23 were pedophiles, 7 were rapists, and 10 were exhibitionists). The treatment with MPA was 400 mg/week for 6 months to 12 years. A control group ($N = 21$) of patients who refused medication were treated with psychotherapy over the same follow-up period. The side effects of MPA were excessive weight gain, malaise, migraine headaches, severe leg cramps, hypertension, various gastrointestinal complaints, and diabetes mellitus. Eighteen percent reoffended while taking MPA, and 35% did so after it was discontinued, compared to a 55% recidivism rate in the control group. The risk factors for reoffense were elevated baseline testosterone levels, previous head injury, and alcohol and drug abuse.

Gottesman and Schubert[60] used low-dose oral MPA in the treatment of the paraphilias. MPA was given at 60 mg/day for 15.33 months in an open trial of seven subjects. Six improved: plasma testosterone levels fell by 50%–75% compared with the baseline. Paraphilic fantasies and behavior were reduced.

LH-RH agonists may also have a role in the treatment of the paraphilias. They produce a "medical or pharmacological castration" in that the hypothalamic-pituitary axis is exhausted and there is a potent inhibition of gonadotropin secretion.[33,77] Rousseau et al.[78] reported on the changes in sexuality of patients with prostate carcinoma who were treated with flutamide (a nonsteroidal true antiandrogen) 750 mg/day in divided doses, in addition to surgical castration. Other patients who did not undergo surgical castration were also treated with flutamide and in addition with an LH-RH agonist, LH-RH ethylamide (D-Trp^6-des-Gly NH$_2$^{10}), administered subcutaneously at 500 µg/day for the first month and then 250 µg/day after this. This latter strategy would be seen as a medical castration. Forty-four patients were studied and their pretreatment sexual functioning was compared to their posttreatment functioning. Before treatment more than 80% of the subjects were having sexual intercourse once a week; more than 50% were able to achieve an erection by erotic imagery or sexual fantasy, and more than 50% had never had any erectile difficulties. After treatment, more than 70% of the subjects noticed a major decline in sexual interest, sexual intercourse was maintained in only 18%, 57% found it impossible to induce an erection by erotic imagery, 19% claimed to be able to maintain an erection for sexual intercourse without full rigidity, 22% had morning erections, and 20% had some level of sexual activity despite significant androgen depletion from both testicular and adrenal origins. Side effects were reported as being minimal.

Rousseau et al.[78] reported a single case of a severe exhibitionist treated with an LH-RH agonist, LH-RH ethylamide [D-Trp[6]-des-Gly NH$_2$[10]]. The dosage was 500 µg/day for 4 weeks and then 250 µg/day for 22 weeks; in addition, flutamide 750 mg/day was administered for the full period of 26 weeks. This extensive androgen blockade ended the exhibitionistic behavior, with a marked decrease in sexual fantasies and sexual activity. Significant side effects were not in evidence. The patient was followed up for 52 weeks. Nine weeks after discontinuing treatment the patient relapsed and started to exhibit and masturbate on a regular basis. There was a sharp increase at week 29 in masturbatory activity, with sexual fantasies returning to baseline or higher levels 7 weeks after discontinuing treatment.

Dickey[79] reported on a treatment resistant-case of paraphilia that had failed to respond to both MPA and CPA. The patient was treated with leuprolide acetate after a failure of treatment with depot MPA and depot CPA. The patient had multiple paraphilias, hebephilia, voyeurism, fetishism, and telephone scatologia. Thibaut et al.[80] reported on the treatment of six paraphilic men treated with the gonadotropin-releasing hormone agonist (GnRHa) triptorelin 3.75 mg/month intramuscularly. Five of the six patients met DSM-III-R criteria for a paraphilia, and one patient had two paraphilias. Pedophilia was the most common paraphilia. The patients were treated by triptorelin 3.75 mg/month concurrently with CPA 200 mg/day for an average of 4.5 months (ranging from 10 days to 12 months). In five patients the deviant sexual behavior was markedly decreased without significant side effects. The follow-up period ranged from 7 months to 3 years. One patient interrupted treatment after 12 months and relapsed in 10 weeks.

Other Pharmacological Agents

An important recent development in the pharmacological treatment of the paraphilias is the use of agents affecting serotonin, such as the serotonin reuptake inhibitors (SRIs). The role of these agents in the treatment of OCDs was presented by Bradford in 1991;[1] In the same paper, Bradford also described the similarities between OCDs and some of the phenomenology of the paraphilias; the possible role of the antilibidinal effects of increased prolactin levels; and the role of 5-hydroxytryptamine in sexual behavior. A detailed open trial in the treatment of pedophilia using an SRI has been undertaken, and the results have been presented. This study includes detailed penile tumescence testing as well as certain biological markers of central serotonin metabolism.[81] Although there is insufficient scientific support at this time to conclude that pharmacological agents affecting serotonin metabolism are indicated for the treatment of a variety of paraphilias, what is available is very supportive of this hypothesis. The importance of this development is twofold:

- The SRIs and other drugs affecting serotonin metabolism are pharmacological agents used by the average psychiatrist when treating depressive syndromes and OCDs. Using these drugs for the treatment of paraphilias is far less threatening to the average psychiatrist than using antiandrogens or hormonal agents. This could therefore result in the average psychiatrist playing a much larger role in the treatment of the paraphilias than has occurred to date.
- Since the onset of the paraphilias occurs in early adolescence with the development of deviant sexual fantasies, and with the

actual deviant sexual behavior occurring after adolescence, an effective treatment that could be safely used in early adolescence is extremely important. Such a treatment could attenuate the development of deviant sexual behavior patterns, which would be a major development in the pharmacological treatment of the paraphilias. Antiandrogens and hormonal treatments have only a limited usefulness in adolescence because of potential side effects, whereas SRIs can be safely used.[1,2,47] In the case of pedophilia the use of SRIs could have an enormous impact in reducing the number of sexual abuse victims in any given society. This is based on the fact that the number of victims of pedophiles increases over time. The potential savings in health care and legal costs are staggering if you consider that the average pedophile can have up to 75 victims over a lifetime of child molesting behavior. Several features of the paraphilias are similar to those of OCDs—for example, onset in adolescence and deviant sexual fantasies that are intrusive and unwanted for the most part (i.e., similar to obsessions). Furthermore, paraphilic behavior can be seen as compulsive.[1,2] This raises an etiological issue as to whether the paraphilias are part of "OCD spectrum disorders" or may even be a kind of impulse control disorder.

Systematic studies of serotonergic agents in the treatment of the paraphilias are currently lacking. There are a number of case reports and some clinical studies of a variety of drugs that look very promising.[82] With few exceptions, the clinical studies do not qualify as open trials. The case reports involving fluoxetine, lithium, buspirone, and clomipramine indicate that they reduce deviant sexual interest in a variety of paraphilias.[1,83–90] There are studies of small numbers of men with paraphilias that show promising results. Kafka[84] showed that paraphilic interest was reduced in 10 subjects with paraphilia and "sexual addiction" who were treated with lithium, fluoxetine, and trazodone. Kafka and Prentky[91] studied 20 subjects (10 with a paraphilia and 10 with a nonparaphilic sexual addiction) in an open trial. The paraphilic group was mainly sexual masochists. No pedophiles were included. There were also a variety of nonparaphilic compulsive sexual behaviors. Of the sample, 95% met DSM-III-R criteria for dysthymic disorder, and 55% for major depression as well. The study duration was 12 weeks with 4-week assessment intervals. There was a 20% dropout rate. Baseline measures compared to outcome at week 12 showed statistically significant improvement in depression and certain sexual behaviors (masturbation, sexual activity, and sexual interest). Stein et al.[3] completed a retrospective review of 13 patients with a paraphilic disorder and nonparaphilic disorder treated with clomipramine, fluoxetine, and fluvoxamine. Five subjects had a paraphilia, five had a nonparaphilic disorder, and nine had comorbid OCD. This was a biased sample, and the OCD appeared to respond, but not the paraphilia in the paraphilic group. In the nonparaphilic group with comorbid OCD and major depression, there was an improvement in 2 of 5 patients. Kruesi et al.[92] treated 15 paraphilic men in a double-blind crossover design of clomipramine versus desipramine. There was a 2-week single-blind period. Eight subjects completed the study and showed some improvement, although no specific difference was noted between clomipramine and desipramine. This is important, because clomipramine is more active at the serotonin receptors. Coleman et al.[93] treated 13 sex offenders with lithium and fluoxetine, with some reduction in deviant interest. Perilstein et al.[94] reported improvement in three patients with paraphilia treated with fluoxetine. Rodenburg et al.[95] reported oxazepam and tryptophan increased deviant sexual activity in three paraphilic men. The disinhibiting effects of oxazepam, among other factors, could explain this result.

Conclusion and Comments

The pharmacological treatment of the paraphilias (including sex offenders) with antiandrogens and hormonal agents is successful in reducing recidivism rates through the reduction of sexual fantasies, sexual drive, sexual arousal, and sexual behavior. The success of the pharmacological treatment approach, as in any treatment approach, depends on the intensive pretreatment evaluation of the person presenting with a paraphilia. This evaluation should include a physiological assessment of sexual arousal, a sex hormone profile, and various questionnaires that measure cognitive distortions and quantify sexual fantasies. The comorbidity of other psychiatric disorders should be established. The degree of alcohol and substance abuse is critical to the ultimate success of treatment. Random urine screening for substances is also a critical component of relapse prevention.

There is some evidence that CPA has a differential effect on the sexual arousal patterns of pedophiles, suppressing the pedophilic arousal and enhancing the arousal toward adult consensual sexual activity. There are questions as to how to use these treatments most effectively and how to select patients most likely to benefit, with a minimum of unwanted side effects. A combined treatment approach using pharmacological and cognitive-behavior treatments should be followed in most paraphilias. If cognitive treatment fails, or if there is evidence of hypersexuality, pharmacological treatments should be used. In the most serious paraphilias such as pedophilia with sexual sadism and sexual sadism directed toward adults (coercive paraphilias) pharmacological treatments should be the primary treatment approach. This may involve "medical castration" through the use of parenteral CPA, MPA, or an LH-RH agonist. There are some medical contraindications to the use of these agents because of the possibility of adverse side effects that are incompletely documented at this time. Freely given informed consent may be problematic where pharmacological treatment is court ordered or is a requirement for parole release. Furthermore, while a person is incarcerated, antiandrogen treatment is not necessary for control and only increases the risk of side effects. Once parole is approved and community reintegration is imminent, then these pharmacological treatments should form part of a community release plan to reduce recidivism.

The need for indefinite ongoing treatment is different with CPA than with LH-RH agonists and MPA. Based on the studies of CPA outlined above, it appears that indefinitely prolonged treatment is not essential to control recidivism. After a treatment period of 6 to 12 months CPA can be gradually tapered off in a significant number of individuals without causing relapses. This does not seem to be true for MPA and LH-RH agonists on the basis of the information that is available. In addition, some individuals are at risk for relapse after discontinuing CPA treatment over a period of time ranging from 6 months to 3 years. When treatment with CPA is discontinued it is important to continue to follow up with an ongoing relapse prevention program. This monitoring allows the earliest sign of potential relapse to be recognized. This is usually the gradual return of sexually deviant fantasies. Part of the relapse prevention strategy is to ensure that the patient is aware of this and can restart CPA treatment at the time the fantasies return. Because of their high risk, some sexually deviant individuals such as sexual sadists need continuous ongoing pharmacological treatment. This is an area of medical research that is underfunded but has extremely high potential for a major impact in sex offender recidivism.

Although more research is necessary to confirm the efficacy of SRIs in large-scale clinical trials, the potential of SRIs in the treatment of the paraphilias and sex offenders is of enormous significance because SRIs give the average general psychiatrist a safe and familiar psychopharmacological tool for the treatment of these problems.

References

1. Bradford JMW: The role of serotonin reuptake inhibitors in forensic psychiatry. Paper presented at the 4th Congress of the European College of Neuropsychopharmacology: The Role of Serotonin in Psychiatric Illness, Monte Carlo, Monaco, October 1991
2. Bradford JMW: Can pedophilia be treated? The Harvard Mental Health Letter 10(9):8, 1994
3. Stein DJ, Hollander E, Anthony DT, et al: Serotonergic medications for sexual obsessions, sexual addictions and paraphilias. J Clin Psychiatry 53:267–271, 1992
4. McElroy SL, Pope SG, Hudson JI, et al: Kleptomania: a report of 20 cases. Am J Psychiatry 148:652–660, 1989
5. Bradford JMW: Organic treatments for the male sexual offender. Behav Sci Law 3(4):355–375, 1985

6. Bremer J: Asexualization—A Follow-up Study of 244 Cases. New York, Macmillan, 1959

6a. Langeluddeke A: Die Entmannung von Sittlich-Keitsver-Brecher. Berlin, de Gruyter, 1963

6b. Cornu F: Katamnesen bein Kastrierten Sittlichkeits-Delinquenten aus Forensisch-Psychiatrischer Sicht. Basel, Switzerland, Karger, 1973

7. Heim N, Hursch CJ: Castration for sexual offenders: treatment or punishment? A review and critique of recent European literature. Arch Sex Behav 8(3):281–304, 1979

8. Le Maire L: Danish experiences regarding the castration of sexual offenders. Journal of Criminal Law, Criminology and Police Science 47:295–310, 1956

9. Ortmann J: The treatment of sexual offenders, castration and antihormone therapy. Int J Law Psychiatry 3:443–451, 1980

10. Sturup GK: Treatment of sexual offenders in Herstedvester, Denmark: the rapists. Acta Psychiatr Scand Suppl 204:5–62, 1968

11. Sturup GK: Castration: the total treatment, in Sexual Behaviors: Social, Clinical and Legal Aspects. Edited by Resnik HLP, Wolfgang ME. Boston, MA, Little, Brown, 1972, pp 361–382

12. Ortmann J: How castration influences on relapsing into sexual criminality among Danish males. Unpublished manuscript, 1984

13. Ortmann J: How antihormone treatment with cyproterone acetate influences on relapsing into sexual criminality in male sexual offenders. Unpublished manuscript, 1984

14. Davidson JM, Smith ER, Damassa DA: Comparative analysis of the roles of androgen in the feedback mechanisms and sexual behavior, in Androgens and Antiandrogens. Edited by Martini L, Motta M. New York, Raven, 1977, pp 137–149

15. Bancroft J: Human Sexuality and Its Problems. Edinburgh, Churchill Livingstone, 1989

16. Wilson JD, Foster DW: Introduction, in Williams Textbook of Endocrinology. Edited by Wilson JD, Foster DW. Philadelphia, PA, WB Saunders, 1985, pp 1–7

17. Liang T, Tymoczko JL, Chan KMB, et al: Androgen action: receptors and rapid responses, in Androgens and Antiandrogens. Edited by Martini L, Motta M. New York, Raven, 1977, pp 77–89

18. Lipsett MB: Regulation of androgen secretion, in Androgens and Antiandrogens. Edited by Martini L, Motta M. New York, Raven, 1977, pp 11–19

19. Mainwaring IP: Modes of action of antiandrogens: a survey, in Androgens and Antiandrogens. Edited by Martini L, Motta M. New York, Raven, 1977, pp 151–161

20. Naftolin F, Ryan KJ, Petro Z: Aromatization of androstenediol in the anterior hypothalamus of adult male and female rats. Endocrinology 90:295–298, 1972

21. Dorner G: Sex-hormone-dependent brain differentiation and reproduction, in Handbook of Sexology II: Genetics, Hormones and Behavior. Edited by Money J, Musaph H. New York, Elsevier, 1977, pp 227–245

22. Bradford JMW, Bourget D: Sexually aggressive men. Psychiatric Journal of the University of Ottawa 12(3):169–175, 1987

23. Bradford JM, McLean D: Sexual offenders, violence and testosterone: a clinical study. Can J Psychiatry 29:335–343, 1984

24. Brown WA, Davis GH: Serum testosterone and irritability in man. Psychosom Med 37:87, 1975

25. Ehrenkranz J, Bliss E, Sheard MH: Plasma testosterone: correlation with aggressive behavior and social dominance in man. Psychosom Med 36:469–475, 1974

26. Kreuz LE, Rose RM: Assessment of aggressive behavior and plasma testosterone in a young criminal population. Psychosom Med 34:321–332, 1972

27. Meyer-Bahlburg HFL, Nat R, Boon DA, et al: Aggressiveness and testosterone measures in man. Psychosom Med 36:269–274, 1974

28. Monti PM, Brown WA, Corriveau DD: Testosterone and components of aggressive and sexual behavior in man. Am J Psychiatry 134(6):692–694, 1977

29. Olweus D, Mattsson A, Schalling D, et al: Testosterone, aggression, physical and personality dimensions in normal adolescent males. Psychosom Med 42:253–269, 1980

30. Persky H, Smith KD, Basu GK: Relation of psychologic measures of aggression and hostility to testosterone production in man. Psychosom Med 40:265–277, 1971

31. Rada RT, Laws DR, Kellner R: Plasma testosterone levels in the rapist. Psychosom Med 38:257–268, 1976

32. Scaramella TJ, Brown WA: Serum testosterone and aggressiveness in hockey players. Psychosom Med 40:262–265, 1978

33. Bradford JMW: Research in sex offenders. Psychiatr Clin North Am 6(4):715–733, 1983

34. Schering AG: Androcur. Berlin, Bergkamen, 1983
35. Neumann F: Pharmacology and potential use of cyproterone acetate. Horm Metab Res 9:1–13, 1977
36. Neumann F, Schleusener A: Pharmacology of cyproterone acetate with special reference to the skin, in The Pharmacology of Cyproterone Acetate, Combined Antiandrogen-Estrogen Therapy, in Dermatology Proceedings of Dianne Symposium. Edited by Vokoer R, Fanta D. Brussels, 1980, pp 19–51
37. Cremonocini C, Viginati E, Libroia A: Treatment of hirsutism and acne in women with two combinations of cyproterone acetate and ethinyloestradiol. Acta European Fertility 7:299–314, 1976
38. Bradford JMW, Pawlak A: Double-blind placebo crossover study of cyproterone acetate in the treatment of the paraphilias. Arch Sex Behav 22:383–402, 1993
39. Laschet U, Laschet L: Psychopharmacotherapy of sex offenders with cyproterone acetate. Pharmakopsychiatrie Neuropsychopharmakologie 4:99–104, 1971
40. Laschet U, Laschet L: Antiandrogens in the treatment of sexual deviations of men. J Steroid Biochem 6:821–826, 1975
41. Davies TD: Cyproterone acetate for male hypersexuality. J Int Med Res 2:159–163, 1974
42. Bancroft J, Tennent G, Loucas K, et al: The control of deviant sexual behavior by drugs: 1. Behavioural changes following oestrogens and anti-androgens. Br J Psychiatry 125:310–315, 1974
43. Cooper AJ: A placebo controlled study of the antiandrogen cyproterone acetate in deviant hypersexuality. Compr Psychiatry 22:458–464, 1981
44. Cooper AJ, Ismail AA, Phanjoo AL, et al: Antiandrogen (cyproterone acetate) therapy in deviant hypersexuality. Br J Psychiatry 120:59–63, 1972
45. Mothes C, Lehnert J, Samimi F, et al: Schering symposium uber sexual deviationen und ihre medikamentose Behandlung. Life Sciences Monograph 2:65, 1971
46. Ott F, Hoffet H: The influence of antiandrogens on libido, potency and testicular function. Schweiz Med Wochenschr 98:1812, 1968
47. Bradford JMW, Pawlak A: Effects of cyproterone acetate on sexual arousal patterns of pedophiles. Arch Sex Behav 22(6):629–641, 1993
48. Bradford JMW, Pawlak A: Sadistic homosexual pedophilia: treatment with cyproterone acetate. A single case study. Can J Psychia-

try 32:22–31, 1987

49. Cooper AJ, Sandhu S, Losztyn S, et al: A double-blind placebo controlled trial of medroxyprogesterone acetate and cyproterone acetate with seven pedophiles. Can J Psychiatry 37:687–693, 1992

50. Cooper AJ, Cernovsky Z, et al: The long-term use of cyproterone acetate in pedophilia: a case study. J Sex Marital Ther 18:292–302, 1992

50a. Horn JH: Die Behandlung von Sexual Delinquenten mit Cyproteron Acetat, in Life Science Monograph 2. Edited by Raspe G. Oxford, UK, Pergamon, 1972, pp 113–122

50b. Baron DP, Unger HR: A clinical trial of cyproterone acetate in sexual deviancy. N Z Med J 85:366–369, 1977

50c. Fahndrich E: Cyproteron acetat in der handlung von sexual deviationen. Dtsch Med Wochenschr 99:234–242, 1974

51. Foote RM: Diethylstilbestrol in the management of psychopathological states in males. J Nerv Ment Dis 99:928–935, 1944

52. Golla FL, Hodge SR: Hormone treatment of sexual offenders. Lancet 1006–1007, 1949

53. Symmers WSC: Carcinoma of breast in trans-sexual individuals after surgical and hormonal interference with the primary and secondary sex characteristics. BMJ 2:82–85, 1968

54. Whittaker LH: Oestrogens and psychosexual disorders. Med J Aust 2:547–549, 1959

55. Field LH: Benperidol in the treatment of sexual offenders. Med Sci Law 13:195–196, 1973

55a. Appelt M, Floru L: Erfahmigen über die beinflussung der sexualität cyproteronacetat. International Pharmacopsychiatry 9:61–76, 1974

55b. Jost F: Klinische beobachtungen und erfahrungen in der behandlung sexueller deviationen mit den antiandrogen cyproteron-acetat. Schweiz Rundsch Med Prax 63:1318–1325, 1974

55c. Jost F: Zur behandlung abnormen sexual verhaltens mit dem antiandrogen cyproteron-acetat. Der Informierte Arzt 3:303–309, 1975

56. Sterkmans P, Geerts F: Is benperidol (RF 504) the specific drug for the treatment of excessive and disinhibited sexual behavior? Acta Neurologica et Psychiatrica Belgica 66:1030–1040, 1966

57. Tennent G, Bancroft J, Cass J: The control of deviant sexual behavior by drugs: a double-blind controlled study of benperidol, chlorpromazine and placebo. Arch Sex Behav 3:261–271, 1974

58. Heller CE, Laidlaw WM, Harvey HI: Effects of the progestational

compounds on the reproductive processes of the human male. Ann N Y Acad Sci 71:649–655, 1958

59. Money J: Discussion of the hormonal inhibition of libido in male sex offenders, in Endocrinology and Human Behavior. Edited by Michael R. London, Oxford University Press, 1968

60. Gottesman HG, Schubert DS: Low-dose oral medroxyprogesterone acetate in the management of the paraphilias. J Clin Psychiatry 54(5):182–188, 1993

61. Meyer WJ, Collier C, Emory E: Depo Provera treatment for sex offending behavior: an evaluation of outcome. Bulletin of the American Academy of Psychiatry and the Law 20(3):249–259, 1992

62. Kiersch TA: Treatment of sex offenders with Depo-Provera. Bulletin of the American Academy of Psychiatry and the Law 18(2):179–187, 1990

63. Berlin FS, Meinecke CF: Treatment of sex offenders with antiandrogenic medication: conceptualization, review of treatment modalities and preliminary findings. Am J Psychiatry 138(5):601–607, 1981

64. Gagne P: Treatment of sex offenders with medroxyprogesterone acetate. Am J Psychiatry 138(5):644–646, 1981

65. Langevin R, Paitich D, Hucker S, et al: The effect of assertiveness training, provera and sex of therapist in the treatment of genital exhibitionism. J Behav Ther Exp Psychiatry 10:275–282, 1979

66. Meyer WJ 3d, Walker PA, Emory LE, et al: Physical, metabolic and hormonal effects on men of long-term therapy with medroxyprogesterone acetate. Fertil Steril 43:102–109, 1985

67. Money J: Use of androgen depleting hormone in the treatment of male sex offenders. Journal of Sex Research 6:165–172, 1970

68. Money JM, Wiedeking C, Walker PA, et al: Combined antiandrogen and counselling program for treatment of 46,XY and 47,XYY sex offenders, in Hormones, Behavior and Psychopathology. Edited by Sachar E. New York, Raven, 1976, pp 105–120

69. Walker PA, Meyer WJ: Medroxyprogesterone acetate treatment for paraphiliac sex offenders, in Violence and the Violent Individual. Edited by Hays JR, Roberts TK, Solway KS. New York, SP Medical and Scientific Books, 1981, pp 353–373

70. Wiedeking C, Money J, Walker PA: Follow up of 11 XYY males with impulsive and/or sex-offending behavior. Psychol Med 9:287–292, 1979

71. Southren AL, Gordon GG, Vittek J, et al: Effect of progestagens on androgen metabolism, in Androgens and Antiandrogens. Edited by Martini L, Motta M. New York, Raven, 1977, pp 263–279

72. Blumer D, Migeon C: Hormone and hormonal agents in the treatment of aggression. J Nerv Ment Dis 160:127–137, 1975

73. Money J, Wiedeking C, Walker P, et al: 47, XYY and 46, XY males with antisocial and/or sex-offending behavior: antiandrogen therapy plus counselling. Psychoneuroendocrinology 1:165–178, 1975

74. Money J: The therapeutic use of androgen-depleting hormone. International Psychiatry Clinics 8:165–174, 1972

75. Cordoba OA, Chapel JL: Medroxyprogesterone acetate antiandrogen treatment of hypersexuality in a pedophiliac sex offender. Am J Psychiatry 140:1036–1039, 1983

76. Wincze WP, Bansal S, Malamud M: Effects of medroxyprogesterone acetate on subjective arousal, arousal to erotic stimulation and nocturnal penile tumescence in male sex offenders. Arch Sex Behav 15:293–305, 1986

77. Rosler A, Witztum E: Treatment of men with paraphilia with a long acting analogue of gonadotropin-releasing hormone. N Engl J Med 338(7):416–422, 1998

78. Rousseau LR, Couture M, Dupont A, et al: Effect of combined androgen blockade with an LHRH agonist and flutamide in one severe case of male exhibitionism. Can J Psychiatry 35:338–341, 1990

79. Dickey R: The management of a case of treatment-resistant paraphilia with a long-acting LHRH agonist. Can J Psychiatry 37:567–569, 1992

80. Thibaut F, Cordier B, Kuhn JM: Effect of a long-lasting gonadotrophin hormone-releasing hormone agonist in sex cases of severe male paraphilia. Acta Psychiatr Scand 87(6):445–50, 199381.

81. Bradford JMW, Greenberg D, Gojer J, et al: Sertraline in the treatment of pedophilia: an open label study (New Research Program Abstracts NR 441). Paper presented at the 148th annual meeting of the American Psychiatric Association, Miami, FL, May 20–25, 1995

82. Fedoroff JP: Serotonergic drug treatment of deviant sexual interests. Annals of Sex Research 6:105–121, 1993

83. Bianchi MD: Fluoxetine treatment of exhibitionism (letter). Am J Psychiatry 147(8):1089–1090, 1990

84. Kafka MP: Successful treatment of paraphilic coercive disorder (a rapist) with fluoxetine hydrochloride. Br J Psychiatry 158:844–847, 1991

85. Emmanuel NP, Lydiard RB, Ballenger JC: Fluoxetine treatment of voyeurism. Am J Psychiatry 148:950, 1991

86. Kerbesian J, Bird L: Tardive syndrome and recurrent paraphilic masturbatory fantasy. Am J Psychiatry 36:155–157, 1991

87. Lorefice LS: Fluoxetine treatment of a fetish (letter). J Clin Psychiatry 52(1):436–437, 1991

88. Pearson HJ, Marshall WL, Barbaree HE, et al: Treatment of a compulsive paraphilic with buspirone. Annals of Sex Research 5:239–246, 1992

89. Wawrose FE, Sisto TM: Clomipramine and a case of exhibitionism. Am J Psychiatry 149:843, 1992

90. Gratzer T, Bradford JMW: Brief communications: A treatment for impulse control disorders and paraphilia: a case report. Can J Psychiatry 40:450–455, 1994

91. Kafka MP, Prentky R: Fluoxetine treatment of non paraphilic sexual addictions and paraphilias in men. J Clin Psychiatry 53:351–358, 1992

92. Kruesi MJP, Fine S, Valladares L, et al: Paraphilias: a double-blind crossover comparison of clomipramine versus desipramine. Arch Sex Behav 21(6):587–593, 1992

93. Coleman E, Cesnik J, Moore AM, et al: An exploratory study of the role of psychotropic medications in treatment of sexual offenders. Journal of Offender Rehabilitation 18:75–88, 1992

94. Perilstein RD, Lipper S, Friedman LJ: Three cases of paraphilias responsive to fluoxetine treatment. J Clin Psychiatry 52:169–170, 1991

95. Rodenburg M, Sheldon L, Owen JA: Sexual disinhibition with L-tryptophan (letter). Can J Psychiatry 37(9):666–667, 1992

CHAPTER 6

Sex Offender Recidivism

The focus in recent years on the recidivism of sexual offenders has been driven by several factors. One concern is the consequences of victimization.[1-5] Another is the enormously high financial costs that sexual offenders cause the community.[6,7] Research into the extent and multiple nature of the paraphilias has also driven this concern.[8,9] A review by Furby and colleagues[10] of the treatment of sex offenders has emphasized research on recidivism and specifically on factors that predict recidivism and treatment outcome.[11-17] This increased focus has heightened awareness of very serious methodological shortcomings in the available information, making it difficult to evaluate the effectiveness of various treatment interventions as well as rates of recidivism in both treated and untreated sex offenders.

In evaluating sex offender recidivism and treatment outcome studies, the following are important considerations:

1. Sexual offenses are grossly underreported, and for this reason most measures of recidivism or treatment outcome are flawed. Whereas rearrest rates and reconviction rates are frequently used, the most accurate, although potentially still flawed, outcome variable may be a combination of these rates and self-reported sexual behaviors that are present in only a few of the reported studies.
2. Reported studies tend to include a variety of sexual offenders and do not differentiate the subjects into subcategories of

paraphilias. The subcategories of pedophilia include heterosexual pedophilia, homosexual pedophilia, and incest. Individuals in these subcategories have different erotic preferences for children and have varying rates of recidivism and treatment outcome. Sex offenders are extremely heterogeneous, and when this is not recognized it is very difficult to make comparisons among studies. Outside of pedophilia, the same problems apply to other paraphilias, such as exhibitionism. Rape, although an important category of sex offender recidivism, is not a paraphilia in the majority of cases. This means that rape often has different precipitants, and therefore rapists have different treatment needs. Treatment outcome is different, and some rapists are untreatable.

3. The most significant methodological problems in recidivism studies are sample selection and study design. Both are problematic in most of the studies, with sample selection being a particularly problematic issue in both treatment outcome and recidivism studies. The majority of studies have used an institutional population, such as penitentiary inmates, selected based on the nature of their criminal activity and the length of the sentence. This bias makes comparisons between studies extremely difficult, and this type of sample is not generally representative of sex offenders or the paraphilias as a whole. Furthermore, sex offenders vary in basic demographics such as age and previous criminal history, including the type of offenses, both sexual and nonsexual. Based on various combinations of these factors alone, different recidivism rates could be expected. In the existing studies this information is often lacking or has not been considered or even reported.

In studies that have differentiated individuals into subcategories such as rapists and pedophiles, problems still exist because of the coexistence of multiple paraphilias.[8,9] The question is what the individual's primary paraphilia is, and whether it has been the target of recidivism studies or treatment.[8,9] For example, pharmacological treatments of the paraphilias clearly have simultaneous impacts on both primary and secondary paraphilias, as do other biological interventions such as surgical castration. Psychological interventions either do not have the same effect on the paraphilias or, if they do, are more inconsistent across various types of psychological treatments.

4. Victim characteristics may also provide a very important way of differentiating recidivism, particularly when they relate to incest perpetrators as a subcategory of pedophilia. The other end of the spectrum would be rapists who target strangers. Victim characteristics have not been considered in a majority of studies, which is a further flaw. Sexually motivated homicides, attempted homicides, and sexually sadistic homicides are also not considered in the existing studies.[18,19]

5. Treatment outcome studies often lack control groups, partly because ethical problems make it very difficult to assign subjects randomly to treatment and nontreatment. Whereas studies employing pharmacological treatments use a double-blind placebo design to compensate for the absence of control groups, psychological interventions are more problematic. Other strategies use "treatment refusers" and treatment dropouts as control groups, but these are limited in their application and raise additional problems.

6. In addition, most of the recent studies are retrospective in design, which also imposes a bias and creates some difficulties in interpretation.

Theoretical Explanations

There have been very few attempts in recent years to conceptualize the theoretical causes of sexual offending. Several theories speculate on the causes from a feminist perspective,[20] as a social phenomenon,[21] as a behavioral phenomenon,[22] and as expressions of various biological factors.[23–29] Hall and Hirschman[30] have taken the various elements of nonbiological models and put forward a model in which sexual aggression is facilitated by the interaction of four motivational factors:

1. Physiological sexual arousal
2. Cognitive distortions that justify sexual offending

3. Negative emotional states
4. Personality or trait variables

These categories interact with multiple factors and have various etiological correlations. For example, the level of pedophilic sexual arousal present in an individual may interact with a cognitive distortion that sex with children is not harmful. This particular individual may also have a history of brain damage leading to poor impulse control with episodes of depression and aggression (as negative emotional states) and may also have personality traits of antisocial personality disorder. Environmental factors are also important, particularly alcohol intoxication, and some recidivism studies have reported a correlation between recidivism and the abuse of alcohol.[10,12,13,15,31]

Recidivism is a complex phenomenon in scientific terms. The following questions illustrate this point: Is a sex offender a recidivist only when he commits the same type of sexual offense, or when he commits any type of sexual offense? What if the offense is nonsexual? Furthermore, parole or probation violation may or may not be an indication of recidivism. In general, the broader the definition of what constitutes recidivism, the higher the expected rate of reported recidivism. Rice et al.[17] showed that rates of recidivism were 31%, 43%, and 58% in a sample of 136 extrafamilial child molesters when recidivism was defined respectively as the reconviction for a sexual offense, reconviction for any violent offense including sexual offenses, and reconviction for any offense. In a similar study of 54 rapists, the recidivism rates were 28%, 43%, and 59%, respectively, using these definitions.[16]

Outcome Measures

There is very little disagreement among researchers that official records of sexual offenses are gross underrepresentations of the actual number of crimes that are committed. Most recidivism studies have relied on official records of arrest or the reconviction rate. This highlights the problems of underreporting, because official arrest rates do not reflect the actual number of acts committed by any paraphilic individual.[8,9,32] In addition, Russell's[33] study of victims involving 900 community women showed that only 2% of intrafamilial (incest) cases, and 6% of extrafamilial cases, of child sexual abuse were reported to the police. Furthermore, the legal process (plea bargaining, for example) creates inconsistencies that may lead to conviction for an offense other than the actual offense.[10] Even self-reporting data are problematic, although such data carry a higher frequency of reported deviant sexual behavior.[8,9] Self-reporting can be profoundly affected by concerns about confidentiality. Kaplan et al.[34] found that subject self-reports admitted to fewer instances of child-molesting behavior than did official records when no guarantee of confidentiality was provided. Self-reported child molestation activity increased by 25% when confidentiality was guaranteed.

Follow-Up Period

Longer follow-up periods show higher rates of reported recidivism.[6,10,13,31,35,36] One of the points that Furby et al.[10] made is that long follow-up periods are needed in order to detect sex offender recidivism, an assertion supported by various studies. For example, Soothill and Gibbens[36] looked at a sample of 178 heterogeneous sex offenders and found that the seriousness of the offenses did not decline even when the period of risk for reoffense exceeded 5 years. Marques et al.[13] concluded from a reanalysis of data collected by Sturgeon and Taylor[37] that a minimum of 5 years at risk was necessary for official records to detect approximately 75% of offenders who recidivated. The study by Hanson and colleagues[35] shows that approximately 10% of a sample of 197 child molesters were reconvicted more than 10 years after release. Some convictions occurred after more than 31 years at risk for reoffense. A recent study by Prentky et al.[38] used a data set of 251 sex offenders, including 136 rapists and 115 child molesters discharged over a 25-year period. They found that both rapists and child molesters were at risk to reoffend many years after their discharge. These researchers defined the category of reoffense as broadly as possible. They found a marked underestimation of recidivism when calculating a simple proportion or percentage of individuals known to have reoffended in the follow-up period. A survival analysis provides a more accurate picture. Using this technique, there was a 53% recidivism or failure rate among extrafamilial child molesters over the 25-year period of being at risk. The rapists were reported as showing a recidivism rate of 39%. This study shows the importance of using the survival analysis technique and defining reoffense in broad terms. The issue of various population samples is not clearly addressed, nor are the effects of treatment.

Other Factors to Consider in Sex Offender Recidivism

As outlined above, some studies report recidivism rates for all offender types grouped together.[14,36,39,40] Other studies have made gross distinctions between offender types such as rapists and all other types of sex offenders.[41] Studies that have differentiated subgroups of sex offenders generally have shown different rates of recidivism for the various subtypes. For example, Marshall and Barbaree[31] found that incest offenders (intrafamilial child molesters) recidivated at about 50% of the rate exhibited by extrafamilial child molesters. Some of the literature makes a broad distinction between the victims based on age, thereby differentiating between child molesters and rapists.[14,16,17,42–44] Further subdivisions are necessary in recidivism studies. Incest perpetrators need to be separated from extrafamilial child molesters.[45–47] Extrafamilial child molesters need to be studied according to whether they are heterosexual, homosexual, or bisexual.[31,43,48–52] There has also been an attempt to subtype rapists and child molesters by sexual arousal.[47,51,53,54] Criminal history has also been investigated.[11,42,49,50,55–57] There have also been studies focusing on various other factors.

The relationship between sexual arousal measured by penile tumescence and sexual offending behavior is stronger in pedophiles than in rapists.[11,44,58-61] In a series of recently completed recidivism studies, the sexual arousal patterns in rapists, extrafamilial child molesters, and incest perpetrators were considered to determine whether they could predict recidivism.[62-64] The sex offenders were followed up for as long as 12 years, with mean survival rates of follow-up of 6.7 years for incest perpetrators, 7.8 years for extrafamilial child molesters, and 7.6 years for rapists. The erections in response to coercive pedophilic stimuli differentiated recidivists among the extrafamilial child molesters, but responses to sexual arousal tests did not differentiate recidivists from nonrecidivists among the rapists or the incest perpetrators. In a large meta-analysis by Hanson and Bussière,[65] the factor most highly correlated to recidivism in over 28,000 sex offenders was erections to children, at a level of $r = .31$. Many factors need to be considered in terms of penile tumescence measurements; some of these are type of stimulus, type of measurement, and the possibility of faking. However, recent studies involving these techniques have shown considerable levels of sensitivity and specificity. Sensitivity is defined as the probability of detecting deviant arousal in offenders, and specificity as the probability of not detecting deviant sexual arousal in nonoffenders. Studies have shown that in detecting rapists, for example, penile tumescence measurements have a specificity of 90% and a sensitivity of only about 60%.[61] In detecting pedophiles, penile tumescence measurements have been shown to have a specificity level of 95% and a sensitivity level of 55% for detecting nonadmitting offenders.[43] Generally the scientific literature supports penile tumescence techniques as a valid method of differentiating sexual deviation in various population samples.

Substance abuse is important in relation to sex offenders. A number of studies have examined alcohol intoxication, alcohol abuse, and alcohol dependency at the time of offense.[23,59,66-69] These studies have shown various rates of alcoholism, ranging between 30% and 50%, with rapists and sexual sadists more likely to have higher frequencies of alcohol consumption than pedophiles. Williams and Finkelhor[45] reported that 57% of incest perpetrators in their study had some problems with alcohol, compared with 44% of a control sample of nonincestuous fathers. More recently, alcoholism has been shown to predict sexual offense recidivism in extrafamilial child molesters,[62] violent recidivism in rapists, and recidivism in incest perpetrators.[63,64] It is not clear how drug abuse may play a role.

Examples of Recidivism Studies

The meta-analysis by Furby et al.[10] considered studies that had to meet strict inclusion criteria. All the recidivism data sources must have included official criminal justice records of rearrest, convictions, or parole violations and have had a defined follow-up period; specifically excluded were studies in which outcome was based solely on self-reporting or on physiological and psychological measures and studies with sample sizes less than 10. Forty-two studies with information from primary sources met the strict criteria for consideration. The recidivism measure was reconviction for another offense. Studies were also divided into two groups based on whether the subjects had received clinical treatment. A large sample of 1,760 offenders released from Atascadero State Hospital in California between 1954 and 1960 were followed up for 1–6 years. The sample was broken down into various subcategories, such as homosexual and heterosexual pedophiles, incestuous and nonincestuous perpetrators, exhibitionists, sexual aggressors, and individuals with other paraphilias.[70] The cumulative recidivism rate through the fifth year was 26.6%. The recidivism rate was 8.7% in the first year; 6.9% in the second year; 5.8% in the third year; 4.8% in the fourth year; 3.2% in the fifth year; and 1.4% in the sixth year. Homosexual pedophiles had a recidivism rate of 34%; heterosexual pedophiles, 21%; incest perpetrators, 10%; exhibitionists, 40%; sexual aggressors, 35%; and a group of others, 46%. The treatment was behavioral.

A pharmacological treatment study by Gagné[71,72] included 87 individuals who were treated for 48 weeks with medroxyprogesterone acetate (MPA) and counseling. The subjects were followed up for 2 years after the completion of the treatment and then were followed up for an additional 2 years. Recidivism was based on official records and self-reporting as "having urges to engage in deviant sexual behavior." According to this extremely broad definition—which includes an urge to act, rather than an actually committed act, as a measure of recidivism—the recidivism rate was 27.6%.

Sturgeon and Taylor[37] studied 260 mentally disordered sex offenders convicted of pedophilia, rape, or incest and treated at Atascadero State Hospital in California. The subjects were discharged after a mean of 19.6 months' incarceration and then followed up for 1–5 years after discharge. The treatment was psychological treatment in groups. The subsequent rate of conviction for a new sexual offense was 15.4%; the rate was 29% for a conviction of any offense. When the sample was broken down into heterosexual and homosexual pedophiles, rapists, and incest perpetrators, the relative recidivism rates were 19.8% for heterosexual pedophiles, 14.6% for homosexual pedophiles, 19.3% for rapists, and 5.3% for incest perpetrators. Also followed up for 1–5 years were 122 individuals convicted of rape, pedophilia, or incest and who served a mean of 54 months in prison and were then paroled. Twenty-five percent of this group received a subsequent conviction for a new sexual offense. In this untreated control group, the heterosexual pedophiles had a recidivism rate of 17.9%; the homosexual pedophiles, 37.5%; the rapists, 29%; and the incest perpetrators, 0%.

Sturup[73] followed up 107 castrated sex offenders and compared them to 58 who were not castrated. The subjects were studied for up to 18 years. The castrated individuals recidivated at a rate of 4.3%. The 58 uncastrated individuals recidivated at a 43% rate—10 times higher than that of the castrated individuals. Gibbens and colleagues[74] studied 170 incest perpetrators (75% were parent-child incest perpetrators and 25% were sibling incest perpetrators) who were incarcerated but untreated. The follow-up period was 12 years. The rate of recidivism was 4% for any sexual offense. These data support the high differential rate of recidivism for incest perpetrators compared with other pedophiles. Gibbens et al.[75] studied 48 untreated heterosexual pedophiles for 24 years after their conviction. Their subsequent rate of recidivism was 29% for sexual offenses and 46% for any criminal offense. The same authors studied another 62 heterosexual pedophiles for 15 years. They found the recidivism rate for sexual offenses was 10%, and for any criminal offense, 35.5%. Gibbens et al.[76] observed 200 rapists, 59 pedophiles, 41 aggressive rapists, and 100 others (who were all untreated sex offenders) for 12 years. The rates of reconviction for the rapists were 7.5% for a sexual offense and 50% for a nonsexual offense; for the pedophiles the rates were 20% for a sexual offense and 63% for a nonsexual offense; for the aggressive rapists, 20% and 85%; and for the other sex offenders, 3% and 28%. Soothill et al.[77] studied 86 convicted rapists (untreated) for 22 years. The subsequent conviction rate for rape was 6%; the conviction rate for rape or other sexual offense was 15%; the subsequent conviction rate for rape, a sexual offense, and an offense of violence to the person was 34%; and the conviction for any serious offense was 49%. Twenty-two men acquitted of rape at the same time were also followed up for 22 years. Their offense reconviction rates, broken down in the same way, were 14%, 29%, 36%, and 57%. Soothill and Gibbens[36] followed up 174 untreated rapists and heterosexual pedophiles for 12–24 years after conviction and reported the subsequent conviction rate for any serious offense was 7.5% in the first year, 9.3% in 2 years, and 48% within 24 years. Soothill et al.[78] followed up 200 untreated convicted rapists for 13 years. The subsequent reconviction rates were 12% for a sexual offense, 19.5% for a violent offense, 27% for a sexual and violent offense, and 49.5% for any serious offense. Fifty-eight men acquitted for rape at the same time had reconviction rates (broken down the same way) of 14%, 29%, 36%, and 57%. These studies give the most reliable statistics for untreated offenders.

Some recent studies[62–64] used better methodology. In a series of studies completed in Ottawa, Canada, the sample consisted of a wide variety of offenders (not just a correctional sample or a sample from a maximum-security hospital, which was preselected) and balanced institutional and community samples. The sample was broken down into extrafamilial child molesters, incest perpetrators, and rapists. The period of follow-up was 12 years, with the mean period of follow-up for the groups being 7.8 years (extrafamilial child molesters), 6.8 years (incest perpetrators), and 7.6 years (rapists). Extensive data were collected on all subjects as part of an assessment at the time of their initial evaluation in a sexual behaviors research clinic. Included in the standardized data were sex hormones, questionnaires, and sexual arousal by a penile tumescence technique. Each patient was assessed using a full psychiatric evaluation and psychological and physiological assessment using objective, scientifically recognized techniques. Offense information was obtained from the Canadian Police Information Center, a national database of both criminal charges and conviction. Furthermore, a survival analysis technique was used. An individual was considered at risk for recidivism only when not incarcerated or in a psychiatric hospital. The first day of eligibility was carefully calculated from the data available. A large sample of sex offenders was studied, and the final samples consisted of extrafamilial child molesters ($n = 192$),[62] incest perpetrators ($n = 251$),[64] and rapists ($n = 85$).[63] These studies of sexual recidivism used a broad definition of reoffense, considered to be any charge or conviction for a sexual offense after the index offense. Violent offense recidivism and general offense recidivism were also documented. Sexual offense recidivism among the extrafamilial child molesters correlated with the guilt scale on the Buss Durkee Hostility Inventory (BDHI),[78a] and the recidivists were in the alcoholism range on the Michigan Alcohol Screening Test (MAST).[78b] The sexual offense recidivists also scored higher on tests of sexual arousal toward children. Violent offense recidivism in this group was associated with a family history of violence and Factor 1 and 2 as well as the Total Score of Psychopathy Check List—Revised (PCL-R).[78c] The physiological sexual arousal also differentiated recidivists from nonrecidivists for violent offenses. Violent offense recidivism was defined as any violent nonsexual offense, and sexual offenses and general offense recidivism were defined as any registered charge or conviction. This cumulative hierarchy was adopted to offset the effects of plea bargaining distortions. General offense recidivism was associated with younger age, less education, drug abuse, previous history of violence, parental substance abuse, family histories of mental illness and violence, removal from parental home before age 16 years, and physical abuse as a child. Sexual offense recidivism in rapists was associated with being removed from the parental home before age 16 and psychological factors such as negativism. Violent offense recidivism in this group was associated with very high scores on the MAST as well as assaultiveness on the BDHI. General offense recidivism was associated with young age, alcoholism, drug abuse, and higher MAST scores. Among the incest perpetrators, sexual offense recidivism was associated with increased MAST scores and higher PCL-R total scores. Violent offense recidivism was associated with increased suspiciousness, higher MAST scores, and higher PCL-R scores. General offense recidivism was associated with individual histories of previous violence and drug abuse; family histories of violence, alcoholism, and criminality; removal from parental home before age 16; and history of childhood physical abuse. On psychological tests these individuals rated themselves higher on assaultiveness and other measures of hostility. They also had higher MAST scores and higher PCL-R scores. Factors most important in predicting future recidivism appear to be the importance of sexual arousal, MAST, PCL-R, and being separated from parents before age 16.

The most significant studies of treated sex offenders involve surgical castration and the antiandrogen cyproterone acetate (CPA). Bremer[79] studied 102 castrates in Norway for a follow-up period of 10 years and found a recidivism rate of 2.9%. Cornu[80] observed 121 castrates in Switzerland for 5 years and found a recidivism rate of 7.4% (4.3% true recidivists). This was compared to 50 men who refused castration and were followed up for 10 years; the rate of reoffense for these subjects was 52%. Langeluddeke[81] studied 932 castrates in Germany with a follow-up period of up to 20 years and found 2.6% were reconvicted of a subsequent sex crime (1% were reconvicted in the first 5 years). Twenty-two percent were convicted of a nonsexual crime. A comparison group of 685 untreated sex offenders (noncastrates) was followed up for 9–20 years. The reconviction rate for this group for a subsequent sex crime was 39.1%.

Antiandrogen treatment studies with CPA are also significant.

The biomedical effects of surgical castration and CPA are very similar. Davies[82] treated 16 sex offenders with CPA in Wales and studied them for 6 months to 3 years, finding a 0% recidivism rate. Fahndrich[83] treated 15 sex offenders with CPA and studied them for 6 months to 3 years. The subsequent sexual offense reconviction rate was 6.7%. Horn[84] treated 33 sex offenders in West Germany and observed them for 1–4.5 years. He found that 6.1% recidivated. Jost[85] treated 11 sex offenders with CPA in Switzerland, followed them up for 3 months to 3 years, and found a 9.1% recidivism rate. Jost[86] treated 10 sex offenders with CPA and followed them up for 1–4 years while they were still in treatment; he found a 10% recidivism rate.

Meta-Analyses of Recidivism Studies

The following are meta-analyses that have been completed: Cox and Daitzman,[87] Blair and Lanyon[88] (23 studies), Kilmann et al.[89] (87 studies), Kelly[90] (32 studies), Finkelhor[91] (10 studies), Borzecki and Wormith[92] (34 studies), Furby et al.[10] (55 studies), and Marshall et al.[93] (4 studies). These meta-analyses cover a large number of studies. The importance of the meta-analyses is that all types of studies, including all types of sex offenders, are considered. In general, most meta-analysis studies had a positive conclusion indicating that treatment appears to be making a positive impact.[94] It is only the Furby et al.[10] study that reports a negative treatment effect. The important issue is that the Furby study refers to North American treatment programs and mostly psychological treatment studies (often group therapy). Furby et al.[10] concluded that 1) there is no evidence that clinical treatment reduces general sex offender recidivism, or whether the effectiveness of such treatment differs in different types of offenders; 2) the longer the follow-up period, the greater the percentage of offenders who commit another crime (not necessarily a sex offense); and 3) there is some evidence that the rate of recidivism may be different for different types of offenders (e.g., incest perpetrators versus heterosexual pedophiles).

Perhaps most important, Furby et al. preselected the least

flawed studies, although the studies were still flawed in various ways. The most important flaw is that in 50% of the studies, subjects were observed for less than 4 years. Furby et al. recommended follow-up periods of at least 10 years. It is important to note that it is principally the biological treatments (castration) that meet these follow-up criteria and that these studies were not North American studies.

Other meta-analyses with their optimistic conclusions ignore the methodological issues and concerns raised by Furby et al.[10] There is no doubt that Furby et al.[10] are excellent researchers, with excellent credentials in statistics and in measuring objective change in a rigorous scientific manner.

A review was also conducted by the U.S. General Accounting Office[95] at the request of the House of Representatives Judiciary Subcommittee on Crime. Information from 22 research reviews on sex offender treatment published between 1977 and 1996 were reviewed and analyzed. Articles were selected through a combination of computerized searches of several databases and by contacting experts. The selected reviews were sent to seven experts in the field to confirm the comprehensiveness of the list. The 22 research reviews covered about 550 studies on sex offenders. Most reviews did not restrict their coverage to a single type of treatment, treatment setting, or offender type. Two focused primarily on a specific treatment setting, one on prison-based treatment programs, and the other on hospital-based programs. Nine focused primarily on cognitive-behavioral approaches, five on organic treatment, and one on psychotherapeutic treatment.

Some of the research reviews concluded that treated offenders had lower recidivism rates than untreated offenders. Others felt that the studies undertaken were so flawed that no firm conclusions could be drawn. Many reviewers were somewhere in between. They tended to conclude that, while some treatment approaches appeared promising, more rigorous research was needed to firmly establish their effectiveness. Even those reviewers who appeared to be among the most positive and optimistic (at least regarding cognitive-behavioral programs) echoed the general sentiment that "there are no conclusive data available from completely method-ologically sound research."[96]

Two meta-analyses and a recidivism study need to be reported here in detail. Hanson and Bussière[65] set out through a meta-analysis to find what factors increased or decreased the risk for recidivism. To be included, studies had to define a group of sex offenders, include a follow-up period, calculate a relationship between an initial characteristic and subsequent recidivism, and record all types of recidivism (sexual, violent, and nonviolent as well as nonsexual recidivism). Eighty-seven studies from six different countries were found, for a total of 28,972 sex offenders with a median follow-up period of 4 years. A common level of predictive accuracy, r, varied from +1 to −1, with a positive value indicating more likely recidivism and a negative value indicating less likely recidivism. The overall recidivism rate for sexual offenses was 13.4%; for nonviolent sexual offenses, 12.2%; and for any recidivism, 36.3%. The strongest predictors of sexual offender recidivism were related to sexual deviance. These included pedophilic sexual preference on phallometric testing ($r = .32$), prior sexual offenses ($r = .19$), age ($r = .13$), early onset of sex offending ($r = .12$), any prior offenses ($r = .13$), and never having been married ($r = .11$). Some general criminological variables were also included. It is important to note that a number of variables were not associated with recidivism, including a history of sexual abuse as a child, substance abuse, and psychopathology (i.e., anxiety and depression). It is important to note also that even the most robust factors cannot be used in isolation to predict recidivism. Combining risk factors in a statistical risk procedure is likely to be of most assistance in the future. Using the first 20 factors from this meta-analysis has been reported as being useful in predicting recidivism, but considerable further research is necessary.

Mary Alexander[97] followed up her 1993 study with a new study involving 81 treatment studies of sex offenders involving 11,350 subjects. Almost all categories of treated sex offenders had recidivism rates less than those of untreated sex offenders (Table 6–1).

The lowest recidivism rates were for juvenile (7.1%) and cas-

Table 6–1. Recidivism among treated versus untreated sex offenders

Category	N	Recidivism (%) Treated	Recidivism (%) Untreated
Juveniles	1,025	7.1	N/A
Rapists	528	20.1	23.7
Child molesters	2,137	14.4	25.8
Exhibitionists	331	19.7	57.1
Not specified		13.1	12.0
Castration subjects		3.3	34.5

Note. N/A, data not available.

trated (3.3%) sex offenders. Relapse prevention was the most successful treatment regardless of subject type. The recidivism rates for juveniles treated were 5.8% for rapists; 2.1% for child molesters; and 7.5% for unspecified offenders. For adults, recidivism rates were 20.1% for rapists; 15.6% for child molesters (female victims); 18.2% for child molesters (male victims); and 4.0% for incest perpetrators. This study shows the success of treatment outcome, and from that standpoint it is an optimistic meta-analysis to be considered in addition to Alexander's previous study.[94,97]

Hall[98] completed a meta-analysis of 12 recent treatment studies including a variety of sex offenders (N = 1,313). The overall recidivism rate for treated sex offenders was .19 compared with .27 for untreated sex offenders. There was a heterogeneous treatment effect across different studies. The effect sizes were larger when base rates of recidivism were higher and when the studies included follow-up of longer than 5 years, included outpatients, and involved cognitive-behavioral or hormonal treatments. Cognitive-behavioral and hormonal treatments were significantly more effective than behavioral treatment.

In our opinion, some conclusions can be made:

- Clearly more treatment outcome studies with matched controls are necessary.

- Follow-up periods of 5–10 years at risk are necessary for definitive conclusions.
- The biomedical treatments show more successful outcomes with long periods of follow-up compared to even the most optimistic of the psychological treatments.

The best chance of a successful outcome would be a combination of biomedical and psychological treatment with a particular emphasis on cognitive and relapse prevention techniques combined with pharmacological treatment.

What the Recidivism Studies Say About Policy-Relevant Questions

Voluntary Versus Mandatory Treatment

Alexander[94,97] shows that mandated treatment appears to have a positive effect in sex offenders, in comparison with voluntary treatment. This makes sense, and mandated treatment should include long-term mandated follow-up in the community, where sex offenders are at risk. A combination of biomedical and psychological treatment should be offered, as well as compulsory relapse prevention groups. Compulsory random urine screening for alcohol and drugs should also be included.

Diagnosis

Generally incest perpetrators, whether treated or not, have lower rates of recidivism than pedophiles and rapists. Generally rapists have the worst prognosis and poorest response to treatment. As rapists do not have a paraphilic disorder in the majority of cases, this may explain this difference.

Offense Class

Offense class is a matter of some debate and is not clearly defined in any of the studies as being important in relation to recidivism.

Biomedical Versus Psychological Treatment

It is very clear that the studies selected by Furby et al.[10] include biomedical treatment studies (surgical castration and CPA) that show very significant improvements in recidivism with biomedical treatment interventions. There are very few psychological treatment studies that compare in terms of outcome, number of subjects, and length of follow-up.

Behavioral Versus Psychodynamic Treatment

There does not appear to be sufficient literature to directly compare these treatments. It is the psychodynamic treatments that are not reported. There is an extensive literature covering cognitive-behavioral, behavioral, and relapse prevention techniques.

The overall impression is that psychodynamic treatments are not reported because they are not successful. The few favorable reports are limited to individual case reports. The result is that cognitive-behavioral and relapse prevention techniques are believed to be more successful and more accepted treatments than psychodynamic treatment approaches.

The final conclusion is that further research is necessary and the treatment approach most likely to have an effect on recidivism is a combined pharmacological, cognitive-behavioral, and relapse prevention approach. Additional pharmacological (biomedical) treatments need to be studied, promoted, and further developed through ongoing research.

References

1. Badgley R, Allard H, McCormick N, et al: Sexual Offenses Against Children, Vol 1. Ottawa, Canadian Government Publishing Centre, 1984
2. Briere JN: Child Abuse Trauma: Theory and Treatment of the Lasting Effects. Newbury Park, CA, Sage, 1992
3. Russell DE: The Secret Trauma: Incest in the Lives of Girls and Women. New York, Basic Books, 1986

4. West DJ: The effects of sex offenses, in Clinical Approaches to Sex Offenders and Their Victims. Edited by Hollins CR, Howells D. Toronto, Wiley, 1991, pp 55–73

5. Manion IG, McIntyre J, Firestone P, et al: Secondary traumatization in parents following the disclosure of extrafamilial child sexual abuse: initial effects. Journal of Child Abuse and Neglect 20(11): 1095–1109, 1996

6. Prentky R, Burgess AW: Rehabilitation of child molesters: a cost-benefit analysis. Am J Orthopsychiatry 60(1):108–117, 1990

7. Freeman-Longo RE, Knopp FH: State-of-the-art sex offender treatment: outcome and issues. Annals of Sex Research 5:141–160, 1992

8. Abel GG, Becker J, Cunningham-Rathner J, et al: Multiple paraphilic diagnoses among sex offenders. Bulletin of the American Academy of Psychiatry and the Law 16(2):153–168,1988

9. Bradford JMW, Pawlak A, Boulet J: The paraphilias: a multiplicity of deviation behaviours. Can J Psychiatry 37:104–108, 1992

10. Furby L, Weinrott MR, Blackshaw L: Sex offender recidivism: a review. Psychol Bull 105(1):3–30,1989

11. Barbaree HE, Marshall WL: Deviant sexual arousal, offense history and demographic variables as predictors of reoffense among child molesters. Behav Sci Law 6(2):267–280, 1988

12. Harris GT, Rice ME, Quinsey VL: Violent recidivism of mentally disordered offenders: the development of a statistical prediction instrument. Criminal Justice and Behavior 20(4):315–335, 1993

13. Marques JK, Day DM, Nelson C, et al: The Sex Offender Treatment and Evaluation Project. Fourth report to the legislature in response to PC 1365. Sacramento, California Department of Mental Health, 1991

14. Pithers WD, Cumming GF: Can relapses be prevented? Initial outcome data from the Vermont treatment program for sexual aggressors, in Relapse Prevention With Sex Offenders. Edited by Laws DR. New York, Guilford, 1989, pp 313–325

15. Quinsey VL, Rice ME, Harris GT: Actuarial prediction of sexual recidivism. Journal of Interpersonal Violence 10(1):85–105, 1995

16. Rice ME, Harris GT, Quinsey VL: A follow-up of rapists assessed in a maximum-security psychiatric facility. Journal of Interpersonal Violence 5(4):435–447, 1990

17. Rice ME, Quinsey VL, Harris GT: Sexual recidivism among child molesters released from a maximum security psychiatric institu-

tion. J Consult Clin Psychol 59(3):381–386, 1991

18. Gratzer T, Bradford JMW: Offender and offense characteristics of sexual sadists: a comparative study. J Forensic Sci 40:450–455, 1995

19. Bradford JMW, Gratzer T: The physiological and psychological characteristics of sexual sadists: a controlled study. Submitted for publication

20. Herman JL: Sex offenders: a feminist perspective, in Handbook of Sexual Assault: Issues, Theories, and Treatment of the Offender. Edited by Marshall WL, Laws DR, Barbaree HE. New York, Plenum, 1990, pp 177–193

21. Malamuth NM, Heavey CL, Linz D: Predicting men's antisocial behavior against women: the interaction model of sexual aggression, in Sexual Aggression: Issues in Etiology, Assessment, and Treatment. Edited by Hall GCN, Hirschman R, Graham JR, et al. Bristol, PA, Taylor and Francis, 1993, pp 63–97

22. Laws DR, Marshall WL: A conditioning theory of the etiology and maintenance of deviant sexual preference and behavior, in Handbook of Sexual Assault: Issues, Theories, and Treatment of the Offender. Edited by Marshall WL, Laws DR, Barbaree HE. New York, Plenum, 1990, pp 209–229

23. Bradford JMW, McLean D: Sexual offenders, violence and testosterone: a clinical study. Can J Psychiatry 29:335–343, 1984

24. Bradford JMW: Organic treatments for the male sexual offender. Behav Sci Law 3(4):355–375, 1985

25. Bradford JMW: Organic treatment for the male sexual offender. Ann N Y Acad Sci 528:193–202, 1988

26. Bradford JMW: The role of serotonin reuptake inhibitors in forensic psychiatry. Paper presented at the 4th Congress of the European College of Neuropsychopharmacology: The Role of Serotonin in Psychiatric Illness, Monte Carlo, Monaco, October 9, 1991

27. Bradford JMW, Pawlak A: Sadistic homosexual pedophilia: treatment with cyproterone acetate. A single case study. Can J Psychiatry 32:22–31, 1987

28. Bradford JMW, Pawlak A: Effects of cyproterone acetate on sexual arousal patterns of pedophiles. Arch Sex Behav 22(6):628–641, 1993

29. Bradford JMW, Pawlak A: Double-blind placebo crossover study of cyproterone acetate in the treatment of the paraphilias. Arch Sex Behav 22:383–402, 1993

30. Hall GC, Hirschman R: Toward a theory of sexual aggression: a

quadripartite model. J Consult Clin Psychol 59(5):662–669, 1991

31. Marshall WL, Barbaree HE: The long-term evaluation of a cognitive-behavioral treatment program for child molesters. Behav Res Ther 26:499–511, 1988

32. Abel GG, Osborn C: The paraphilias: the extent and nature of sexually deviant and criminal behavior. Clinical Forensic Psychiatry 15(3):675–687, 1992

33. Russell DEH: The incidence and prevalence of intrafamilial and extrafamilial sexual abuse of female children. Child Abuse Negl 7:133–146, 1983

34. Kaplan MS, Abel GG, Cunningham-Rathner J: The impact of parolees' perception of confidentiality of their self-reported sex crimes. Annals of Sex Research 3:293–304, 1990

35. Hanson RK, Steffy RA, Gauthier R: Long-term recidivism of child molesters. J Consult Clin Psychol 61(4):646–652, 1993

36. Soothill KL, Gibbens TCN: Recidivism of sexual offenders. British Journal of Criminology 18(3):267–276, 1978

37. Sturgeon VH, Taylor J: Report of a five-year follow-up study of mentally disordered sex offenders released from Atascadero State Hospital in 1973. Criminal Justice Journal 4(31):31–63, 1980

38. Prentky RA, Lee AFS, Knight RA, et al: Recidivism rates among child molesters and rapists: a methodological analysis. Law Hum Behav 21(6):635–659, 1997

39. Berliner L, Miller LL, Schram D, et al: The Special Sex Offender Sentencing Alternative: a study of decision making and recidivism. Report to the Washington state legislature. Journal of Interpersonal Violence 10(4):487–502, 1995

40. Dwyer SM, Rosser BRS: Treatment outcome research cross-referencing a six month to ten-year follow-up study on sex offenders. Annals of Sex Research 5:87–97, 1992

41. Tracy F, Donnelly H, Morgenbesser L, Macdonald D: Program evaluation: recidivism research involving sex offenders, in The Sexual Aggressor: Current Perspectives on Treatment. Edited by Greer JG, Stuart IR. New York, Van Nostrand Reinhold, 1983, pp 198–213

42. Bard LA, Carter CL, Cerce DD, et al: A descriptive study of rapists and child molesters: clinical, and criminal characteristics. Behav Sci Law 5(2):203–220, 1987

43. Freund K, Blanchard R: Phallometric diagnosis of pedophilia. J Consult Clin Psychol 57(1):100–105, 1989

44. Malcolm PB, Andrews DA, Quinsey VL: Discriminant and predictive validity of phallometrically measured sexual age and gender preference. Journal of Interpersonal Violence 8(4):486–503, 1993

45. Williams, Finkelhor D: The characteristics of incestuous fathers: a review of recent studies, in Handbook of Sexual Assault: Issues, Theories, and Treatment of the Offender. Edited by Marshall WL, Laws DR, Barbaree HE. New York, Plenum, 1990, pp 231–255

46. Freund K, Watson R, Dickey R: Sex offenses against female children perpetrated by men who are not pedophiles. Journal of Sex Research 28(3):409–423, 1991

47. Marshall WL, Barbaree HE, Eccles A: Early onset and deviant sexuality in child molesters. Journal of Interpersonal Violence 6(3):323–336, 1991

48. Freund K, Watson RJ: The proportions of heterosexual and homosexual pedophiles among sex offenders against children: an exploratory study. J Sex Marital Ther 18(1):34–43, 1992

49. Marshall WL, Barbaree HE, Butt J: Sexual offenders against male children: sexual preferences. Behav Res Ther 26(5):383–391, 1988

50. Marshall WL, Barbaree HE, Christophe D: Sexual offenders against female children: sexual preferences for age of victims and type of behaviour. Canadian Journal of Behavioural Science 18(4):424–439, 1986

51. Murphy WD, Haynes MR, Stalgaitis SJ, et al: Differential sexual responding among four groups of sexual offenders against children. Journal of Psychopathology and Behavioral Assessment 8(4):339–353, 1986

52. Prentky RA, Knight RA, Rosenberg R, et al: A path analytic approach to the validation of a taxonomic system for classifying child molesters. Journal of Quantitative Criminology 6(3):231–257, 1989

53. Barbaree HE, Marshall WL: The role of male sexual arousal in rape: sex models. J Consult Clin Psychol 59(5):621–630, 1991

54. Barbaree HE, Serin RC: Role of male sexual arousal during rape in various rapist subtypes, in Sexual Aggression: Issues in Etiology, Assessment and Treatment. Edited by Hall GCN, Hirschman R, Graham JR, et al. Bristol, PA, Taylor and Francis, 1993, pp 99–114

55. Baxter DJ, Barbaree HE, Marshall WL: Sexual responses to consenting and forced sex in a large sample of rapists and nonrapists. Behav Res Ther 24(5):513–520, 1986

56. Hall GCN: Criminal behavior as a function of clinical and actuarial

variables in a sexual offender population. J Consult Clin Psychol 56(5):773–775, 1988

57. Prentky RA, Knight RA, Sims-Knight JE, et al: Developmental antecedents of sexual aggression. Dev Psychopathol 1:153–169, 1989

58. Barbaree HE: Stimulus control of sexual arousal: its role in sexual assault, in Handbook of Sexual Assault: Issues, Theories, and Treatment of the Offender. Edited by Marshall WL, Laws DR, Barbaree HE. New York, Plenum, 1990, pp 115–142

59. Baxter DJ, Marshall WL, Barbaree HE, et al: Deviant sexual behaviour: differentiating sex offenders by criminal and personal history, psychometric measures, and sexual response. Criminal Justice and Behavior 11(4):477–501, 1984

60. Serin RC, Malcolm PB, Khanna A, Barbaree HE: Psychopathy and deviant sexual arousal in incarcerated sexual offenders. Journal of Interpersonal Violence 9(1):3–11, 1994

61. Lalumiere ML, Quinsey VL: The sensitivity of phallometric measures with rapists. Annals of Sex Research 6:123–138, 1993

62. Firestone P, Bradford JMW, McCoy M, et al: Prediction of recidivism in court-referred child molesters. Submitted for publication in Sexual Abuse: a Journal of Research and Treatment

63. Firestone P, Bradford JMW, McCoy M, et al: Recidivism in court-referred extra-familial child molesters. Submitted for publication

64. Firestone P, Bradford JMW, Greenberg DM, et al: Prediction of recidivism in incest offenders. Journal of Interpersonal Violence 14 (March), 1999

65. Hanson RK, Bussière MT: Predictors of Sexual Offender Recidivism: A Meta-analysis (User Report No 1966–04). Ottawa, Department of the Solicitor General of Canada, 1996

66. Hucker S, Langevin R, Wortzman G, et al: Neuropsychological impairment in pedophiles. Canadian Journal of Behavioural Science 18(4):440–448, 1986

67. Rada RT, Laws DR, Kellner R: Plasma testosterone levels in the rapist. Psychosom Med 38(4):257–267, 1976

68. Rada RT, Laws DR, Kellner R, et al: Plasma androgens in violent and nonviolent sex offenders. Bulletin of the American Academy of Psychiatry and the Law 11(2):149–158, 1983

69. Allnutt S, Bradford JMW, Greenberg D, et al: Comorbidity of alcoholism and the paraphilias. J Forensic Sci 41:134–139, 1995

70. Frisbie LV, Dondis EH: Recidivism Among Treated Sex Offenders (California Mental Health Research Monograph No 5). Sacramento, CA, State of California Department of Mental Hygiene, 1965

71. Gagné P: Treatment of sex offenders with medroxyprogesterone acetate. Am J Psychiatry 138(5):644–646, 1981

72. Gagné P: Pretreatment prognosis predictors in sexual deviants. Paper presented at the Congress on Criminal Justice, Vancouver, BC, 1985

73. Sturup GK: Sexual offenders and their treatment in Denmark and other Scandinavian countries. International Review of Criminal Policy 4:1–19, 1953

74. Gibbens TCN, Soothill KL, Way CK: Sibling and parent-child incest offenders. British Journal of Criminology 18:40–52, 1978

75. Gibbens TCN, Soothill KL, Way CK: Sex offenses against young girls: a long-term record study. Psychol Med 11:351–357, 1981

76. Gibbens TCN, Way CK, Soothill KL: Behavioral types of rape. Br J Psychiatry 130:32–42, 1977

77. Soothill KL, Jack A, Gibbens TCN: Rape: a 22 year cohort study. Med Sci Law 16(1):62–69, 1976

78. Soothill KL, Way C, Gibbens TCN: Rape acquittals. Modern Law Review 43:159–172, 1980

78a. Buss AH, Durkee A: An inventory for assessing different kinds of hostility. Journal of Consulting Psychology 21:343–349, 1957

78b. Selzer ML: The Michigan Alcohol Screening Test: the quest for a new diagnostic instrument. Am J Psychiatry 127(12):1653–1658, 1971

78c. Hare RD: The Hare Psychopathy Checklist—Revised Manual. Toronto, ON, MultiHealth Systems Inc., 1990.

79. Bremer J: Asexualization—a follow-up study of 244 cases. New York, Macmillan, 1959

80. Cornu F: Catamnestic Studies on Castrated Sex Delinquents From a Forensic Psychiatry Viewpoint [in German]. Basel, Karger, 1973

81. Langeluddeke A: Castration of Sexual Criminals [in German]. Berlin, Degruyter, 1963

82. Davies TD: Cyproterone acetate for male hypersexuality. J Int Med Res 2:159–163, 1974

83. Fahndrich E: Cyproteronacetat in der Behandlung von Sexualdeviationen bei Männern. Dtsch Med Wochenschr 99:234–242, 1974

84. Horn JH: The treatment of sexual delinquents with cyproterone ace-

tate, in Life Sciences Monograph 2. Edited by Raspé G. New York, Pergamon, 1972, pp 113–123

85. Jost F: Klinische Beobachtungen and Erfahrungen, in Der Behandlung Sexueler Deviationen mit dem Antiandrogen Cyproterone-Acetate. Schweiz Rundsch Med Prax 63:1308–1325, 1975

86. Jost F: Zur Behandlung Abnormen Sexualverhaltens mit dem Antiandrogen Cyproterone-Acetate, 1971–1975. Der Informier-tearzt 3:303–309, 1975

87. Cox DJ, Daitzman RJ: Behavioral theory, research and treatment of male exhibitionism, in Progress in Behavior Modification. Edited by Hersen M, Eisler RM, Miller PM. New York, Academic Press, 1979, pp 63–116

88. Blair CD, Lanyon RI: Exhibitionism: etiology and treatment. Psychol Bull 89:439–463, 1981

89. Kilmann PR, Sabalis RF, Gearing ML, et al: The treatment of sexual paraphilias: a review of the outcome research. Journal of Sex Research 18(3):193–252, 1982

90. Kelly RJ: Behavioral reorientation of pedophiliacs: can it be done? Clin Psychol Rev 2:387–408, 1982

91. Finkelhor D: A Source Book on Child Sexual Abuse. Beverly Hills, CA, Sage, 1986

92. Borzecki M, Wormith JW: A survey of treatment programmes for sex offenders in North America. Canadian Psychology/Psychologie Canadienne 28:30–44, 1987

93. Solicitor General of Canada: The Management and Treatment of Sex Offenders: Report of the Working Group Sex Offenders Treatment Review. Ottawa, Minister of Supply and Services, 1990

94. Alexander MA: Sex offender treatment: a response to the Furby, et al. 1989 quasi-meta-analysis. Paper presented at the Association for the Treatment of Sexual Abusers Conference, Boston, MA, November 1993

95. U.S. House of Representatives, Committee on the Judiciary, Subcommittee on Crime, Report to the Chairman. Research results inconclusive about what works to reduce recidivism. Washington, DC, U.S. General Accounting Office, June 1996

96. Marshall WL, Anderson D: An evaluation of the benefits of relapse prevention programs with sexual offenders. Unpublished manuscript

97. Alexander MA: Sex offender treatment probed anew. Unpublished document, 1997

98. Hall GCN: Sexual offender recidivism revisited: a meta-analysis of recent treatment studies. J Consult Clin Psychol 63:802–809, 1995

CHAPTER 7

Frequently Asked Questions

1. What would be required reading for a general psychiatrist who is considering treating patients with paraphilias?

A number of texts can be recommended, including the following:

1. *Sourcebook of Treatment Programs for Sexual Offenders.* Edited by W. L. Marshall, Y. M. Fernandez, S. M. Hudson, et al. New York, Plenum, 1998
2. *Sexual Deviance: Theory, Assessment, and Treatment.* D. Richard Laws and William O'Donohue. New York, Guilford, 1997
3. *The Sex Offender:* Volume 1, *Corrections, Treatment and Legal Practice,* and Volume 2, *New Insights, Treatment Innovations and Legal Developments.* Edited by Barbara K. Schwartz and Henry R. Cellini. Kingston, NJ, Civic Research Institute, 1997
4. *Sexual Deviation,* 3rd Edition. Edited by Ismond Rosen. Oxford, UK, Oxford University Press (Oxford Medical Publications), 1996
5. *Handbook of Sexual Assault.* D. R. Laws. Edited by H. E. Barbaree and William L. Marshall. New York, Plenum, 1990
   Covers all the major topics.
6. *Relapse Prevention With Sex Offenders.* D. Richard Laws. New York, Guilford, 1989
   Explains the relapse prevention model as it applies to sex offenders.

7. *Pedophilia: Biosocial Dimensions.* Jay R. Feierman. New York, Springer-Verlag, 1990

    Includes a broad range of topics such as ethology, evolution, hormones, and neuroendocrinological factors contributing to pedophilia.

8. *Juvenile Sex Offending: Causes, Consequences, and Correction.* Edited by Gale D. Ryan and Sandy L. Lane. San Francisco, CA, Jossey-Bass, 1991

    One of the few books dealing specifically with adolescent sex offenders.

9. *Changing Inappropriate Sexual Behavior: A Community-Based Approach for Persons With Developmental Disabilities.* Dorothy M. Griffiths, Vernon L. Quinsey, and David Hingsburger. Baltimore, MD, Paul H. Brookes, 1989

    One of the few texts available regarding developmentally delayed offenders.

10. *Treating Child Sex Offenders and Victims.* Anna C. Salter. Newbury Park, CA, Sage Publications, 1988

    Includes many commonly used paper-and-pencil tests for evaluating sex offenders.

2. Are there methods of gathering objective evidence of sexual interest for use with the courts or for treatment purposes?

There are three objective means of determining sexual interest in sex offenders: penile plethysmography, visual reaction time assessment, and polygraphs. Plethysmography and visual reaction time assessmentpresent the patient with stimuli specific to various deviant sexual interests and record the patient's response during such presentations. Polygraphy is used to gather information regarding the validity of the suspected offender's self-report. None of the three methods provides a level of validity that meets any of the prevailing standards required for admissibility in court as scientific evidence. However, proper use of these methods can provide the clinician with valuable information regarding offenders' sexual interests, which can then be incorporated into the psychiatrist's total evaluation of the patient.

3. Which cases may be suitable for diversion from the criminal justice system from a therapeutic standpoint?

Cases of incestuous child molestation that do not involve intercourse with the child are generally appropriate for diversion from the criminal justice system. An extensive literature indicates that, irrespective of the treatment modality, recidivism rates in this population are exceedingly low. However, the therapist should recommend diversion only when the perpetrator is out of the home, involved in treatment, and under intensive supervision by his or her probation officer. When the perpetrator has been involved with children under age 14 as well as adolescents ages 14–17 in activities that involve touching (such as fondling) and nontouching (such as exhibitionism or voyeurism) against females and males, this is called the crossing of diagnoses. Individuals who cross into more categories of victims and behaviors are at higher risk to reoffend. Perpetrators who admit to their offense(s) and accept responsibility for their actions are more suitable for diversion than are those who deny their actions or attempt to place the blame for their behavior either on their victim(s) or others. Also, those who have demonstrated compliance with therapy before adjudication are more suitable for diversion.

4. What are the essential elements of a good sex offender treatment program in a community? How do you go about finding one?

A good community sex offender treatment program has evaluation and treatment for a variety of problematic areas usually seen in sex offenders. These components include the assessment of inappropriate sexual interests (that may lead to sex offending), cognitive distortions or rationalizations (that perpetrators use to justify their inappropriate behavior), victim empathy (that identifies whether the perpetrator appreciates the consequence of his or her behavior on the victim), assertive skills and anger management (common problematic areas with sex offenders), social skills (another common deficit of sex offenders), relapse prevention (identifies risk

factors for reoffense and how to effectively manage them), drug
and alcohol problems (alcoholism especially is correlated with sex
offending), marital difficulties (seen before and after sex offending
behavior), developmental delays, intellectual limitations, attention
deficit disorder and organic brain disease (sometimes seen as an
antecedent to sex offending), and time management (sex offenders
frequently offend when they have time on their hands). Good sex
offender treatment programs can be found by contacting organizations that specifically deal with sex offender evaluation and treatment such as the Association for the Treatment of Sexual Abusers,
10700 Southwest Beaverton-Hillsdale Highway, Suite 26,
Beaverton, OR 97005–3035 (telephone 503-643-1023) or The Safer
Society Program and Press, P. O. Box 340, Brandon, VT 05733 (telephone 802-247-3142). These organizations should be able to direct
you to treatment programs in your vicinity. Select programs if possible that have seen at least 50 sex offenders per year, since such
programs generally have a more integrated approach that includes
cognitive-behavior treatment and medication intervention if indicated.

**5. A prison would like to set up a program for sex offenders.
What should be minimally (or optimally) a part of the program
that would be a useful expenditure of funds?**

Optimally, a prison program would provide all the services of an
outpatient treatment program. However, implementing a psychiatric service within a prison setting can be difficult. An inpatient
program should normally satisfy the following criteria:

- The staff should confront the sex offender with all of the available information that led to his conviction so as to be certain that
  there is consistency between his appreciation of his sex crime
  and his own self-reporting of the offense.
- The staff should understand and apply the relapse prevention
  model as it is applied to sex offenders so that the offender is
  knowledgeable about what constitutes the appropriate elements
  of treatment.

- Every effort should be made to incorporate the offender's family so that they too are aware of all of the evidence regarding the perpetrator's inappropriate behavior. When the family is knowledgeable, it makes it easier to design outpatient treatment once the offender has left the prison setting.
- Offenders should be taught how to access the outpatient treatment programs in proximity to where they would be living and how to work with their probation or parole officer to ensure that the requirements of probation or parole are met.

6. John Doe has been accused of sexual assault. He denies the charges. With what degree of certainty can you tell his attorney that he is an incest offender, a pedophile, or an aggressive rapist? What test should normally or minimally be done before drawing any conclusions?

a) If the victim is Doe's 5-year-old daughter. Assuming the accusation is that he molested his 5-year-old daughter, one should complete a psychiatric clinical interview, administer paper-and-pencil tests to determine whether he self-reports arousal to children, administer a measure of cognitive distortions frequently seen with pedophiles, and review all of the records surrounding the incident available from the criminal justice system (if available) and from the patient's lawyer. The clinician should also obtain an objective measure of sexual interest in children (using visual reaction time or plethysmography), gather a social history from those in his environment who can provide additional information regarding his behavior around the child and children, and, if acceptable to his attorney, arrange for a polygraph. Some individuals molest their daughters because they have pedophilic interest and the daughter happens to be a child living at home who is easily accessible. Many incestuous involvements, however, do not involve deviant sexual interest toward children but are related to drug and alcohol abuse, isolation from appropriate sexual partners, the impact of divorce, or organic brain disease. If the individual is a pedophile with chronic sexual attraction to young girls, it may be possible to ascertain this arousal pattern by the objective measurements. However, no objective measurement could ever determine whether (assuming the individual was a pedophile) he has involved himself with his own daughter. Objective measures should not be used in a court of law to determine such issues.

b) If the victim is a 13-year-old boy. The clinical evaluation should proceed as described in (a). If the alleged victim is a 13-year-old boy, objective measures will be more effective at determining sexual interest, because objective measures have always been more valid when the alleged victim is male rather than female. Once again, however, such measures should not be taken into court to prove or disprove whether the individual has actually been sexually involved with the 13-year-old boy.

c) If the victim is a 23-year-old woman. Finally, if the alleged victim is a 23-year-old woman, it is unlikely that objective measures will be particularly helpful at showing and demonstrating arousal to 23-year-olds. Instead, the patient should be presented with stimuli reflecting a rape or sexual assault or sadistic assault on an adult woman, to determine if the alleged perpetrator is responsive to stimuli depicting a sexual assault. Even then, however, if the client is responsive to such cues, these could not be used to prove one way or the other whether the patient has actually attempted to rape or has raped the woman. Polygraph examination can be very useful with individuals accused of inappropriate sexual behavior with adult victims to help determine the validity of their self-report.

Assessment of inappropriate sexual interests, including clinical interviews, paper-and-pencil tests, and psychophysiological measures are designed to identify individuals who are in need of specialized therapy. These techniques were not designed, nor should they be used, for attempting to determine guilt or innocence regarding specific allegations.

7. John Doe has been convicted of sexual assault. What factors should a psychiatrist use in a report for a court or parole board assessing safety for release?

a) If the victim is his 5-year-old daughter. When the victim is the offender's 5-year-old daughter, the psychiatrist should ascertain the degree to which the patient's report of what he has done is consistent with the investigative information. The greater the consistency, the less the risk. If John Doe has many faulty cognitions and cognitive distortions that justify and rationalize his reason for sexually assaulting his 5-year-old daughter, he is at greater risk to reoffend. If he has been involved with male and female children less than age 14 years and ages 14–17 years, inside and outside the family—that is, if the crossing into various categories of deviant behavior is greater—the risk is greater. If John Doe's family, particularly his sexual partner, denies his involvement with his daughter, he is at greater risk to reoffend. The number of involvements with his daughter may not be a very good predictor of his risk for reoffense, as one might imagine.

b) If the victim is a 13-year-old boy. If the victim of John Doe's sexual assault is a 13-year-old boy, the risk for recidivism will be greater than if the victim were his daughter, since recidivism for incest is low. The other factors that increase the risk of recidivism will hold for the 13-year-old boy as well.

c) If the victim is a 23-year-old woman. When the conviction is for the sexual assault of a 23-year-old woman, one also needs to determine if Mr. Doe has an antisocial personality disorder (which increases recidivism considerably), whether he has had multiple charges of sexual assault of adult females, and whether his report of the assault conflicts with that of the victim. All of these factors are suggestive of increased risk for recidivism.

Another significant factor to consider in all of these cases is whether the perpetrator has received specialized sex offender therapy (as described above) while in prison, and how well he did in that treatment.

8. John Doe has been convicted of sexual assault, has served his sentence, and is about to be released. What treatment program

and/or drugs and in what progression would you prescribe to deal with repetitive urges after release from prison?

All convicted sex offenders should receive cognitive-behavior treatment with a strong relapse prevention element unless there is an exceedingly powerful reason to forgo such treatment. If Mr. Doe's urges to reoffend begin to accelerate, the frequency of cognitive-behavior treatment should be increased and the psychiatrist should consider the addition of a selective serotonin reuptake inhibiting drug (SSRI) to reduce the individual's sexual drive (as a side effect of the SSRI). If the repetitive urges continue in spite of cognitive-behavioral treatment and administration of SSRIs or if the potential victim is quite young, or if the sexual assault behavior includes physical force against the victim, or if Mr. Doe has sadistic interest, the psychiatrist should consider adding medroxy-progesterone acetate (Provera), in an oral or injectable form, and if this is unsuccessful, the psychiatrist should consider the use of leuprolide acetate (Lupron). Lupron, however, should be used cautiously for the first few weeks because there will be a temporary increase in sexual drive, as Lupron works as an agonist for luteinizing hormone–releasing hormone. During this latter time the patient should be hospitalized or closely supervised by family.

9. Who should get antiandrogens? Who should not?

Antiandrogens are typically given to sex offenders if a less intrusive treatment has proved ineffective, if their victims are quite young, if they report poor control over their urges, or if the damage done to victims has been extensive. Antiandrogens have generally been used in excessively high doses under the assumption that castrate levels of testosterone should be reached before considering reduction of the dose. However, castrate levels produce serious side effects that frequently lead the sex offender to discontinue medication. Antiandrogens, in the past, have been administered in a depot (injectable and long-acting) form. The depot form, however, reduces compliance with treatment. The psychiatrist should first consider the administration of antiandrogens by mouth and at a relatively lower dose than that reported in the literature (a maximum dose might be in the neighborhood of 200 mg by mouth daily). The goal of administering antiandrogens is to reduce the tremendous pressure and sex drive that some (but not all) sex offenders have. The goal, however, should not be to eliminate sexual interest completely.

Antiandrogens should be given with care to sex offenders with liver damage, obesity, gallbladder disease, diabetes, and a prior history of thrombophlebitis and to those who have a low frequency of sexual offending.

10. What offender groups are not treatable?

The major scientific problem in evaluating who is or is not responsive to treatment is that the mental health professions have not made a concerted effort to provide treatment for sex offenders. As a consequence, many studies of treatment outcome rely on data collected 15–20 years ago at a time when cognitive-behavior treatment, relapse prevention, and drug intervention were not used. Even recent studies do not provide good measures of treatment efficacy because whatever treatment is provided within the prison setting has not been extended to the community after release and has not been coupled with a cooperative effort with parole and probation officers to ensure proper monitoring and therapy maintenance.

The more appropriate question is who is more difficult to treat, and under what level of supervision, rather than who cannot be treated. At the present time we have only tentative answers to these questions. The category of individuals who are most difficult to treat includes those who deny that they have any paraphilic interests and/or that they have carried out any inappropriate sexual behavior. Denial is a common trait of perpetrators, and treatment programs should provide specific therapy to help perpetrators work through their denial. However, when the individual continues to deny inappropriate sexual interests or behavior, he is not able to substantially benefit from therapy and should be considered a treatment failure and still at high risk to the community.

Perpetrators whose behavior tends to occur at a high frequency with minimal or no consequences are difficult to treat because they generally lack motivation to change. Therefore, transvestites, fetishists, public masturbators, exhibitionists, and voyeurs, as a group, will tend to have higher recidivism rates. If arrested at all, these perpetrators tend to be charged with misdemeanors and are often treated "lightly" by the criminal justice system. As a result, they are less likely to enter treatment or to be motivated to do so. Although they are a more difficult group to treat and are more likely to reoffend while in treatment, they tend to present minimal risk of significant injury to the community and thus can often be treated on an outpatient basis. This is especially true when these individuals are treated with SSRIs concomitantly with their cognitive-behavioral therapy.

The comorbid existence of brain pathology, substance and alcohol abuse, developmental delays, and learning disabilities make treatment more difficult. Also, individuals who have concomitant problematic personality disorders are more difficult to treat because the personality disorder may interfere with the individual's ability to comply with treatment requirements. For example, rapists of adult victims who do not appear to have the characteristics of a paraphilia are often difficult to treat because there is generally a strong antisocial personality component to their sex offending.

A final means of distinguishing those expected to have higher recidivism is to identify individuals who have more than one area of inappropriate sexual interest. A tendency to have multiple categories of paraphilic interests and/or behavior is called the *crossing of diagnoses*. The greater the crossing of diagnostic categories, the more problematic treatment becomes. In general, the paraphilias in order of greatest to least likelihood of crossing of diagnosis are sadism, public masturbation, incestuous pedophilia involving boys, fetishism, masochism, voyeurism, nonincestuous pedophilia involving females, exhibitionism, nonincestuous pedophilia involving boys, transvestism, frottage, incestuous pedophilia involving girls, and rape of adult females.

Although few perpetrators are "untreatable," some require higher levels of supervision while undergoing treatment, such as supervised living, probation, intensive probation or house arrest, hospitalization, or incarceration. Although these generalities provide guidelines for determining risk for reoffense, each case should be evaluated on its individual merits.

CHAPTER 8

Policy Recommendations

How many sex offenders have a mental disorder? Is it appropriate to involuntarily commit "sexual predators" to psychiatric hospitals as mentally ill and dangerous? What should be the standards for commitment? What kinds of treatment are appropriate, and where and when should they be administered? What is the role of involuntary treatment? What, if anything, should be done with dangerous sex offenders who have completed their sentences? Should they be treated differently than other convicted felons who have served their sentences and may be just as likely to recidivate if released back into the community? These questions have resulted in a complicated and contentious debate for the past 50 years.

Since 1990, the debate has been escalated by the passage in some states of "sexual predator" statutes permitting a new form of psychiatric civil commitment for an indeterminate period following completion of a prison sentence. These sexual predator laws echo an earlier generation of "sexual psychopath" statutes enacted in the mid-20th century, many of which were later repealed. They were, however, held to be constitutional by the U.S. Supreme Court.[1,2] The sexual predator laws differ from the sexual psychopath statutes in a number of ways, but most importantly in the fact that the sexual psychopath statutes generally resulted in hospitalization as an alternative to prison rather than following the completion of a prison sentence. Just as the repeal of the sexual psychopath statutes was frequently triggered by released offenders repeating crimes, the passage of the sexual predator statutes in many cases has been precipitated by convicted offenders repeating sexual offenses shortly after their release from prison. Despite objections by the American Psychiatric Association (APA), the U.S. Supreme Court in *Kansas v. Hendricks* upheld the constitutionality of one of these statutes in June 1997.[3]

The current wave of statutes can best be understood as a response to several changes in the criminal justice system that have resulted in convicted felons being released back into the community prematurely and repeating heinous crimes. These changes reflect the trend to have "determinate" or fixed sentences for convicted felons rather than "indeterminate" sentencing, which allowed prison officials flexibility in determining an offender's release date. Although recidivism rates for convicted felons are high in general, sex offenders have always had especially high visibility because of the nature of their crimes and the fact that the majority of victims are women or children.

Psychiatric practice and public sector treatment programs are heavily affected by the proliferation of these new commitment laws, and the profession has an obligation to understand and be able to provide professional advice to legislatures regarding the nature of such legislation. In order to do so effectively, an understanding of the nature of the disorders, the status of current treatment, and the availability of such treatments is essential. In addition, it is important to consider how the new proposals may affect the integrity of existing treatment programs, as well as the cost and cost-effectiveness of these new efforts. A major goal of the Task Force report is to educate the profession and the public about the current understanding of sexual disorders and developing treatments for sex offenders.

After summarizing current knowledge regarding the diagnosis and treatment of violent sex offenders, the Task Force presents its conclusions and recommendations regarding this group of disorders and the role of psychiatry in the treatment process.

Diagnosis and Treatment of
Dangerous Sex Offenders:
A Summary of Current Knowledge

Diagnosis

The paraphilias consist of a group of disorders characterized by recurrent intense sexual urges and fantasies. Affected persons suffer clinically significant distress or impairment of social, occupational, or other areas of functioning associated with these urges. Various systems have been developed for classifying such disorders. Distinctions based on the nature or age of the target are common—rapists, pedophiles, zoophiles. Pedophiles, for example, either act on or are distressed by their fantasies about or activities with prepubescent children. The amount of aggression that may be involved is another distinction (e.g., sadism). Some features of these disorders are akin to obsessions and compulsions. This observation is strengthened by the response of some paraphilias to pharmacological agents used in the treatment of obsessive-compulsive disorders. The fact that paraphilias, like the substance abuse disorders, may lead to criminal behavior is not in itself a proper basis for refusing to offer available and appropriate treatment.

Earlier studies suggested that most persons suffering from paraphilia displayed behaviors characteristic of only one of these disorders. More recent studies have demonstrated that there is extensive crossover between the paraphilic disorders. The disorders and behaviors in which crossover is very limited are transsexualism, ego-dystonic homosexuality, rape of adult females, and female incest pedophilia. It is not surprising that transsexualism and ego-dystonic homosexuality have a low rate of crossover, as DSM-IV does not list them as paraphilias. Female incest pedophilia, likewise, may be more the result of the easy availability of the female child rather than a recurrent, compulsive, paraphilic interest.

Whether or not any rapist has a paraphilia represents a controversial issue in the research literature. DSM-IV has not classified paraphilic rapism as a mental disorder. Some researchers believe that a small group of rapists have diagnostic features similar to those with other paraphilias. The ability to make the diagnosis with a sufficient degree of validity and reliability remains problematic. In addition, other research has shown that many rapes are not the product of primary sexual interests but rather represent an exercise in power and control. In a study looking at a variety of demographic and criminal factors in several samples of incarcerated offenders, the authors concluded, "There is little difference between rapists and either property or violent offenders. . . . The offender group with which rapists differed most were the other sex offenders."[4]

Recidivism

It is difficult to draw definitive conclusions from the existing research data on sex offender recidivism because of substantial limitations in research design, length of follow-up, gross underreporting of sexual offenses, and divergent measures of the criterion variable. However, it does appear that, in general, incest offenders, whether treated or not, have lower rates of recidivism than pedophiles and rapists. Generally, rapists have the worst prognosis and the poorest response to treatment.

Treatment

The biomedical treatments (surgical castration and administration of cyproterone acetate—an antiandrogen) appear to result in significant reduction in recidivism rates. However, the existing literature does not show involuntary medication to be effective as the sole treatment. Behavioral and psychodynamic treatments have not been compared in controlled studies. The psychodynamic treatments tend to be described in individual case reports. There is extensive literature covering cognitive-behavior and relapse prevention techniques. The most reasonable conclusion at this time is that cognitive-behavior and relapse prevention techniques are more successful and more accepted treatments than psycho-dynamic treatment, although treatment efficacy is controversial for every approach.

Clearly, further research is necessary. The best that can be said at present is that the treatment approach most likely to have an effect on recidivism is a combined pharmacological, cognitive-behavior, and relapse prevention approach.

> **Conclusions and Recommendations on Research and Training**
>
> Although sound epidemiological data do not exist, it is clear that a significant number of people have paraphilic disorders, that these disorders cause substantial personal and social distress, and that only a small proportion of those individuals receives treatment in either community settings or correctional institutions. Although scientific understanding of the paraphilic disorders has improved in recent years, the societal investment in research has not been commensurate with the need for new knowledge relating to the diagnosis and treatment of persons with these disorders and the effects of therapeutic interventions on recidivism. Training programs for psychiatrists and other mental health professionals have devoted inadequate attention to the assessment and treatment of persons with paraphilic disorders.
>
> The Task Force recommends increased investment in research on paraphilic disorders and in the clinical training of psychiatrists and other mental health professionals regarding assessment and treatment of persons with those disorders.

Legal Control of Dangerous Sex Offenders: The Propriety of Civil Commitment

The medical model of civil commitment is fundamentally paternalistic. In general, involuntary hospitalization is believed to be warranted when necessary to protect individuals whose ability to recognize their need for treatment is impaired by serious mental illness.[5] Under the APA's Model Guidelines, civil commitment is permitted only if a person has a "severe mental disorder," which is defined as "an illness, disease, organic brain disorder or other condition that substantially impairs the person's thought, perception of reality, emotional process, or judgment, or substantially impairs behavior as manifested by recent disturbed behavior." By requiring a severe mental disorder, the APA intends to reserve involuntary treatment for only a small class of seriously disturbed persons for whom psychiatric intervention is most appropriate. As explained in the commentary to the model law, "substantial impairment means more than transitory disorientation or an isolated phobia or sensitivity. It ordinarily entails broad deterioration in the structure, content or integration of one of the cognitive or affective processes indicated." Severe mental disorders will also result in severe disability and typically intense emotional distress. Even if a disorder is capable of producing such impairments, to qualify as a mental illness for purposes of involuntary hospitalization, such hospitalization must be medically justifiable.[6]

Society has recognized the importance of civil commitment and treatment of the mentally ill. Courts have made important distinctions between civil commitment and other forms of detention, such as criminal incarceration, based on the paternalistic nature of psychiatric intervention. For example, those facing criminal incarceration are constitutionally entitled to strict procedural protections (e.g., trial by jury, the right to remain silent), and the state must prove that punishable acts occurred beyond a reasonable doubt. On the other hand, civil commitment proceedings may incorporate relaxed procedural protections and lower standards of proof. The essentially paternalistic character of civil commitment is reflected in the fact that the statutory predicates for involuntary hospitalization are typically established by expert psychiatric opinion.

Sexual predator commitment statutes are *not* fundamentally paternalistic. These statutes reflect a backlash against determinate sentencing reform and are devised to extend the punishment of sex offenders and to protect society. To evade constitutional protections against ex post facto laws, to impose indeterminate confinement, and to take advantage of relaxed procedural safeguards, drafters of sexual predator commitment statutes have attempted to cloak their quasi-punitive intent in the language of medical commitment.

These commitments are also very expensive, because they require maximum-security facilities. In the states where such confinements have been implemented, costs have varied between $60,000 and $130,000 per year for each person, not including the cost of the legal proceedings. States have not always provided additional funding for these programs and have thereby drained resources from existing mental health services. Family and consumer organizations have objected, noting the danger other patients face when hospitalized with predators and decrying the stigma that naturally attaches to the association with this population.

> In the opinion of the Task Force, sexual predator commitment laws represent a serious assault on the integrity of psychiatry, particularly with regard to defining mental illness and the clinical conditions for compulsory treatment. Moreover, by bending civil commitment to serve essentially nonmedical purposes, sexual predator commitment statutes threaten to undermine the legitimacy of the medical model of commitment. In the opinion of the Task Force, psychiatry must vigorously oppose these statutes in order to preserve the moral authority of the profession and to ensure continuing societal confidence in the medical model of civil commitment.

The Misuse of Diagnostic Terminology and Methods

The formulation of psychiatric diagnoses is the prerogative of the psychiatric profession. Revising the diagnostic nomenclature and updating diagnostic criteria are core professional responsibilities that—rightfully—involve substantial investment of psychiatrists' time and effort. It is the special province of psychiatry to undertake these tasks and to base judgments regarding nomenclature and criteria on research findings and therapeutic goals.

Psychiatrists have recognized that only persons with severe mental disorders should be subject to civil commitment. Diagnostic skills are called on to ascertain whether substantial impairments and broad deterioration of cognitive or affective processes are present. Moreover, psychiatrists must exercise their judgment regarding whether hospitalization is medically justifiable (see the APA Model Civil Commitment Law).[7] Psychiatric judgment on these matters protects against the use of civil commitment for inappropriate reasons. For example, in some countries, corrupt governments have wielded the machinery of civil commitment to punish dissidents. In the United States, civil commitment has sometimes been misused to confine social deviants.

In contrast to the true medical model of commitment, the sexual predator commitment laws do not base the criteria for the "diagnosis" of sexual predator on psychiatric research or therapeutic findings. Typically, sexual predator status is based on a vague and circular determination that an offender has a "mental abnormality" that has led him to engage in repeated criminal behavior. Because the element of mental abnormality is so vague, it does little or nothing to qualify the requirement for criminal acts. Thus, these statutes have the effect of defining "mental illness" in terms of criminal behavior. Indeed, the Washington legislature's findings with regard to that state's statute expressly disavowed the idea that the target group has a serious mental illness. As explained in the statute, the target group is made up of individuals "who do not have a mental disease or defect that renders them appropriate for the existing involuntary treatment act."[8]

In the opinion of the Task Force, the sexual predator commitment laws establish a nonmedical definition of what purports to be a clinical condition without regard to scientific and clinical knowledge. In so doing, legislators have used psychiatric commitment to effect nonmedical societal ends that cannot be openly avowed. In the opinion of the Task Force, this represents an unacceptable misuse of psychiatry.

Treatment of "Sexual Predators"

Under the medical model, civil commitment is justified when effective treatment is provided.[9] Therefore, an individual can be involuntarily hospitalized only if potentially beneficial treatment is available for his or her disorder (see the APA Model Civil Commitment Law).[5] Under the sexual predator commitment statutes, because mental illness is not defined in legitimate terms, there is no assurance that those who are committed have any mental disorder at all. Based on anecdotal evidence, it appears that many of those who are committed do not suffer from a mental disorder; some may have a paraphilia; and others may have personality disorders.

Although a body of research indicates that some types of paraphilias may be treatable, this research for the most part concerns patients who are treated voluntarily. In characterizing those treated in these studies as "voluntary," the Task Force recognizes that many individuals accepted treatment as a result of some element of legal coercion. Many of these patients participated in diversion programs or sought treatment as a result of criminal prosecution. Nonetheless, the Task Force recognizes that many sex offenders choose *not* to participate in diversion programs and refuse available treatment. Thus, there is no evidence regarding the efficacy of available treatments for the group of patients who have little or no motivation for treatment. Moreover, no evidence supports the notion that persons with paraphilias can be treated successfully without their cooperation. Indeed, as discussed in an earlier section, to date there is no clear basis for making the claim that treatment of any class of patients with paraphilias will result in lower rates of recidivism.

There is no evidence that the sexual predator commitment statutes are being applied only to those who may benefit from treatment. To the contrary, there is ample anecdotal evidence that those committed as sexual predators cannot benefit from treatment. In many cases, the lack of treatment prospects appears to flow from the lack of a legitimate psychiatric diagnosis. In other instances, it appears that offenders who suffer from paraphilias cannot be treated because they are uncooperative. Regardless of the reason, it is the opinion of the Task Force that confinement without a reasonable prospect of beneficial treatment of the underlying disorder is nothing more than preventive detention and violates the norms of the medical model.

The Task Force recognizes that the U.S. Supreme Court has upheld the constitutionality of these statutes and that many states are likely to enact them. It is important to emphasize, however, that several justices were willing to uphold the Kansas statute only on the assumption that it would be applied to patients with genuine psychiatric disorders, such as paraphilias, and that a bona fide therapeutic effort would be undertaken. If a state chooses to adopt such a statute, the criteria for mental disorder should explicitly include a diagnosed DSM-IV disorder involving significant impairment of impulse control relating to sexual behavior. Moreover, the statute should guarantee the availability of adequate treatment opportunities to patients who are willing to take advantage of them. Finally, any stand-alone civil commitment statute for sex offenders should apply *only* to individuals who have been found, beyond a reasonable doubt, to have committed a sexually violent offense. Whether the commitment scheme is in lieu of criminal conviction and sentencing or is imposed after expiration of a criminal sentence, a necessary condition for commitment as a sex offender should be proof of the predicated sexual offense beyond a reasonable doubt. The state should ensure that these new sex offender commitment laws do not erode the boundaries or safeguards of ordinary civil commitment. Specifically, a term of ordinary civil commitment should not be extended solely on the basis of concern that a patient will commit a sexual offense if the person does not otherwise meet the criteria for ordinary civil commitment.

Conclusions and Recommendations on Civil Commitment

Societal concerns about the need for punishment and incapacitation of dangerous sex offenders should be met through customary sentencing alternatives within the criminal justice system and not through involuntary civil commitment statutes.

Treatment of Dangerous Sex Offenders Within the Criminal Justice System

Ultimately, problems with determinate sentencing should be corrected by rethinking the appropriate terms of imprisonment for dangerous sex offenders. Even during the few years since the Washington statute was enacted, there has been a nationwide trend toward prescribing long terms of confinement, often mandatory, for offenders who have committed violent sexual offenses.

It is unfortunate that state legislatures have focused on sexual predator commitment laws while voluntary treatment programs within correctional settings have remained unfunded or underfunded. Offenders who may have treatable problems, either paraphilias or other conditions that may contribute to criminal behavior—such as drug and alcohol abuse—are not receiving needed care. The Task Force recommends that states establish adequately funded programs within the correctional system that are based on current clinical knowledge. Such programs can be implemented through a variety of legal models, including diversion and indeterminate sentencing.

Sex offenders should have an opportunity to participate in treatment programs while serving criminal sentences whether or not such participation has any bearing on the nature and length of their sentences. Participation in such programs should not be mandatory.

Various models may be considered. For example, therapeutic incentives for sex offenders with paraphilic disorders could be established with "special track" indeterminate sentencing arrangements for offenders who elect to participate and who are found clinically suitable. Under such a model, early release may be based in part on evidence of a positive response to treatment efforts.

Regardless of whether such special tracks are created, the Task Force believes that better services need to be made available in correctional settings. Evaluation and treatment efforts should not be postponed to the eve of completion of prison sentences. As with individuals with substance abuse disorders, adequate treatment of those with sexual disorders during and after incarceration is important. Diversion programs, mandated treatment as a condition of probation or parole, and other models are worthy of consideration.

Conclusions and Recommendations on the Treatment of Sex Offenders Within the Criminal Justice System

Legislatures and correctional agencies genuinely interested in providing therapeutic opportunities for dangerous sex offenders as a means of reducing the rate of recidivism should establish adequately funded programs within the correctional system that are based on current clinical knowledge. Such programs can be implemented through a variety of legal models, including diversion and indeterminate sentencing.

Sex offenders should have an opportunity to participate in treatment programs while serving criminal sentences whether or not such participation has any bearing on the nature and length of their sentences. Participation in such programs should not be mandatory.

Legislatures interested in developing therapeutic dispositional incentives for sex offenders with paraphilic disorders should consider "special track" indeterminate sentencing arrangements for offenders who elect to participate and who are found clinically suitable. Under such a model, an administrative body similar to the bodies that now review and monitor insanity acquittees could determine the conditions of confinement and release.

"Chemical Castration" Laws

In 1996, California passed a law that predicates release from prison for certain classes of sex offenders on "chemical castration" with antiandrogenic agents.

Antiandrogenic agents have an appropriate role in the treatment of patients, including some types of convicted sex offenders, who have been selected by psychiatrists following appropriate diagnostic assessment. Patients who have been selected for treatment based on clinical criteria, including diagnosis of a disorder indicating treatment, absence of disorders contraindicating use of these agents, and motivation for treatment, may benefit from treatment with antiandrogenic agents.

Identification for treatment based solely on offense improperly equates psychiatric diagnosis with criminal behavior. Many inmates in the class of offender will not have a diagnosis of a psychiatric disorder or one that would justify treatment with these agents. Certainly not all patients who have been prescribed antiandrogens have engaged in criminal behavior. Laws treating criminal conduct as equivalent to a mental disorder serve to stigmatize psychiatric disorders and discourage treatment seeking.

The criminal justice system undermines the integrity of psychiatry by designating "treatment" based on legal, rather than clinical, criteria. Some eligible offenders, even though they do not have a psychiatric disorder, may choose to undergo "treatment" to obtain release from prison. Psychiatrists may be pressured to provide treatment to these inmates inappropriately. The use of chemical castration misappropriates psychiatric knowledge in another way. The bill characterizes the treatment as "in addition to any other punishment prescribed for that offense." This raises confusion about the role of psychiatry and seems to endorse the view of psychiatrists as primarily agents of punishment and social control.

Finally, the appropriation by the criminal justice system of antiandrogenic agents for purposes of social control represents a serious misunderstanding of therapeutic interventions and the basis of their efficacy. Antiandrogenic agents have been used effectively by psychiatrists who have selected patients on clinical grounds. Often, other types of treatment, such as cognitive and behavioral therapies, must be coadministered to achieve therapeutic results. Inmates selected on the basis of offense category are not likely to have the same response to administration of these agents. Moreover, many inmates will not be motivated to change their behavior and cannot be expected to cooperate with the medication regimen. Androgenic agents, such as the widely available testosterone patch, can readily counteract the hormonal effects of antiandrogenic agents, rendering the "treatment" ineffective.

Conclusions and Recommendations on
"Chemical Castration" Laws

Laws that predicate release from prison on "chemical castration" by
surgery or antiandrogenic agents for broad classes of sex offenders
are objectionable because they are not based on adequate diagnostic
and treatment considerations and because they improperly link
medical treatment with punishment and social control.

Notes

1. Minnesota ex rel Pearson v Probate Court, 309 US 270 (1940)
2. Specht v Patterson, 386 US 605 (1967)
3. Kansas v Hendricks, 521 U.S. 346; 117 S. Ct. 2072 (1997)
4. Alder C: The convicted rapist: a sexual or violent offender? Criminal Justice and Behavior 11:157–177 (1984)
5. The APA Model Civil Commitment Law suggests the following criteria for involuntary patients: 1) the person is suffering from a severe mental disorder; and 2) there is a reasonable prospect that his disorder is treatable at or through the facility to which he is to be committed and such commitment would be consistent with the least restrictive alternative principle; and 3) the person either refuses or is unable to consent to voluntary admission for treatment; and 4) the person lacks capacity to make an informed decision concerning treatment; and 5) as a result of the severe mental disorder, the person is a) likely to cause harm to himself or to suffer substantial mental or physical deterioration, or b) likely to cause harm to others.
6. American Psychiatric Association: Guidelines for Legislation on the Psychiatric Hospitalization of Adults. Am J Psychiatry 140:672–679, 1983 [as approved by the Assembly of District Branches, October 1982; and by the Board of Trustees, December 1982]
7. The APA Model Civil Commitment Law includes an additional requirement that is relevant to the severity of mental disorder. Under the APA model, in order to qualify for commitment, a mentally ill individual must be incompetent to make the hospitalization decision.
8. Wash Rev Code § 71.09.010

9. For individuals who are so incapacitated by untreatable mental illness that they cannot care for themselves, commitment may be justified on general paternalistic grounds, rather than on therapeutic grounds.

Index

*Page numbers printed in **boldface** type refer to tables or figures.*